FOURTEEN HEALING OILS

YOU CAN'T LIVE WITHOUT AND MORE!

Super Dirt Cheap Healers You Just Have To Know About Today!

...boost the immune system, even though it is not completely understood how it works!

Brought dramatic relief to inflammation and stiff joints caused by rheumatoid arthritis!

Seriously ill cancer patients were treated... 90 days, tumors gradually receded!

The antiseptic powers... are GIGANTIC...!

... remove toxins like mercury from the body!

far less heart disease than Americans, ... they drink, smoke, consumed more saturated fat...!

is a POTENT CLEANSER - DETOXIFIER!

...period of approximately 90 days, tumors gradually receded!

TOP SECRET! Includes 01 More SUPER HEALER You Just Have To Know About Today!!

100% Satisfaction Guarantee

JOSEPH A. LAYDON JR.

"Fourteen Healing Oils You Can't Live Without And More!"

UPDATED: 211851C April 2023 (Thursday)

Published By Joseph A. Laydon Jr.

Website: https://www.survivalexpertblog.com

E-Mail: wwwsurvivalexpert@yahoo.com

MOST IMPORTANT NOTE: The individual *"Fourteen Healing Oils You Can't Live Without And More"* is a compilation from my already published 46 *Anytime Anywhere Survival Newsletters (AASN)*.

Copyright & Disclaimer

IRISAP DISCLAIMER STATEMENT

The author of *"Fourteen Healing Oils You Can't Live Without And More!"* and owner of Intensive Research Information Services And Product(s) (IRISAP) is exercising his right under the First Amendment to self-publish and co-author this informational product to better educate the public with respect to being more self-reliant Anytime Anywhere. The author is publishing this information based upon his *"intensive research"* and his experiences. Author is demonstrating through this Survival Book how to become a bit more self-reliant when it comes to Health Survival.

This Survival Book is designed to help the reader become more aware of the unique applications of Alternative Therapies employing Oils.

The information within this Survival Book is for educational purposes only. Professional advice from *"qualified medical professionals "* is ALWAYS and HIGHLY recommended. Advice is neither implied nor intended. IRISAP and authors\writers of resource materials are not responsible for the purchaser's and third party activities and is in no way responsible for sickness or death or successes.

THE PURCHASER OF THIS SURVIVAL BOOK IS SOLELY RESPONSIBLE FOR THIRD PARTY DISCLOSURE AND RESPONSIBLE FOR THEIR ACTIONS AND ANY PRIVATE OR PROFESSIONAL ACTIONS TAKEN FROM THIS INFORMATIONAL PRODUCT.
This Special Report is Copyrighted and VIOLATORS WILL BE PROSECUTED!

If the consumer DISAGREES with ANY portion of this DISCLAIMER STATEMENT, the consumer MUST immediately (upon receipt) return this entire informational product for a full refund.

Table Of Contents

Contents

Dedication!

This Survival Book - *"Fourteen Healing Oils You Can't Live Without And More!"* is dedicated to all the past, present and future sickly and dead patients who put their total 100% trust in conventional medicine of drugs and surgery and failed to overcome their sickly maladies.

There are better alternatives to the multitudes of sickly therapies of drugs used in conventional medicine.

There are more than 60 Alternative Therapies. 60 Alternative Therapies that are worthy of your attention. The 667-page Gettysburg Program found at **www.survivalexpertbooks.com** is where the Gettysburg Program and other data can be found concerning Alternative Therapies used throughout the world and throughout history.

This Survival Book - *"Fourteen Healing Oils You Can't Live Without And More!"* barely, barely, barely touches all those 60+ Alternative Therapies. I highly encourage you to see all my Survival Books at:

https://www.survivalexpertblog.com/52-survival-books/

Introduction

Welcome and thank you for getting *"**Fourteen Healing Oils You Can't Live Without And More!**"* where you'll find real healthy survival tricks that compliment any alternative health knowledge you may already possess. Learn about these *"healthy healing oils"* so *You're Ready Anytime Anywhere.*

Somebody in your family household has to be the Survival Expert - even when it comes to alternative healthcare when conventional medicine has failed. Somebody has to be the Survival Expert, why not you? And here's a good start so *You're Ready Anytime Anywhere!*

I HIGHLY encourage you to visit **https://www.survivalexpertblog.com/52-survival-books/** and see three books that complement this Survival Book:

- *"**99+ International Cancer Preventers, Cancer Fighters, Cancer Killers And More!**"*
- *"**99+ International Heart Attack Preventers, Heart Attack Fighters, Heart Attack Killers And More!**"*
- *"**99+ International Diabetes Preventers, Fighters, Killers And More!**"*

Again, thank you for getting this Survival Book.

IMPORTANT NOTE: *"**Fourteen Healing Oils You Can't Live Without and More!**" is not in alphabetical order. I encourage you to read this Survival Book multiple times so *You're Ready Anytime Anywhere!*

"Fourteen Healing Oils You Can't Live Without And More!"

Here are *"Fourteen Healing Oils You Can't Live Without And More"* that are worthy of your attention. OK, let's start with *Healing Benefits Of Shark Liver Oil*.

NOTE: These *"Fourteen Healing Oils You Can't Live Without And More* <u>**are not in alphabetical order**</u> and are direct quotes from several Anytime Anywhere Survival Newsletters from the *2012 Ultra-Advanced Anytime Anywhere Survival Program TOTAL Package (2012 U-AAASPTP)*.

"Italy and Greece have lower heart disease and stroke"

"...help protect arteries and blood vessels by significantly lowering bad-type blood cholesterol (LDL)"

"...brought dramatic relief to inflammation and stiff joints caused by rheumatoid arthritis."

"used for centuries for common colds, flues, minor aches and inflammation"

"the consumption of as little as one or two fish dishes per week may be of preventive importance in relation to coronary heart disease."

"People in the Mediterranean have been noted to develop far less heart disease than Americans"

"Mediterranean groups had lower death rates, longer life expectancies in Greece than in any other European or North American country despite their high tobacco consumption, low exercise level and modest health-care system"

"...researchers have successfully blocked both migraine headaches and kidney disease..."

"...ameliorating, healing, reversing, preventing: accelerated wound healing, allergies, asthma, atherosclerosis, brain tumors including other cancers, Candida fungus..."

"...successfully blocked both migraine headaches and kidney disease..."

"...rates high for keeping blood pressure in a healthy range. Jichi Medical School in Japan have shown that levels of "good" HDL cholesterol were high among Japanese..."

"Oregano could turn into the next wonder drug."

"I have to tell you about the healing benefits of ____ remarkable healing and health enhancing oils!"

"I decided this oil was going to be my healer, my banishment for this cussing toothache pain from hell"

"It provides something that enables men to bear hard stress and continue to do hard labor without deteriorating. It particularly affects physical endurance and heart response."

"has anti-bacteria, anti-fungal, and anti-viral agents"

"it was found to be 48 times more potent than fish oil"

"According to Dr. Judith Wurtman, principal investigator at MIT, the high protein in fish, namely the amino acid tyrosine, may boost the brain neurotransmitters norepinephrine and dopamine, which energizes your mind and makes you feel more alert."

Shark Liver Oil

Olive Oil

Omega-3 Fatty Acids

Castor Oil

Flaxseed Oil

Oil Of Oregano

Clove Oil

Wheat Germ Oil

Coconut Oil

Panaseeda Oil

Fish Oil

Tea Tree Oil

Turpentine Oil

Krill Oil

The Super Healing Effects Of Oil Pulling

Weight-Loss Oils To The Rescue

LOSE FAT BY EATING FATS

The Mediterranean Diet

BONUS HEALING

Unadvertised BONUS BONUS For YOU

OK, let's get started with *"Healing Benefits Of Shark Liver Oil."*

"Healing Benefits Of Shark Liver Oil!"

Initially a Scandinavian folk medicine, Shark Liver Oil has been used for centuries for common colds, flues, minor aches and inflammation. Shark Liver Oil has now drawn the attention of scientist, doctors and health enthusiast all around the world!

Its early research focused on enhancing the immune system, radiation treatment protection, and reduction in the mortality rate of cancer patients. Health enthusiast have noted benefits of Shark Liver Oil such as ameliorating, healing, reversing, preventing:

- accelerated wound healing
- allergies
- asthma
- atherosclerosis
- brain tumors including other cancers
- Candida fungus
- Colds
- chronic fatigue syndrome
- cosmetic decline
- flu...

What gives Shark Liver Oil its healing benefits? Shark Liver Oil contains squalene, omega-3 oils (EPA & DHA), alkylglycerols (AKGs) and other substances, but for this Survival Book, we'll talk about the special healing ingredients.

What is squalene?

An element of shark oils, squalene is generally related to Vitamin A. Some shark livers contain as much as 65% squalene by weight. Used in the cosmetic industry, it is noted to benefit the skin with the use of skin moisturizers.

What are Alkylglycerols (AKGs)?

AKGs support the requirements of the white blood cell (immune system). Oil-based chelating agents, AKGs remove toxins like mercury from the body.

Benefits of AKGs are noted to be:
- anti-bacterial
- anti-fungal
- anti-inflammatory (arthritis)
- arterial walls become more elastic
- asthma
- heavy metals are removed via oil-based chelating.
- immune system enhancement
- inhibits blood clots
- lowering LDL cholesterol (bad cholesterol)
- promotes vasodilatation (lowers blood pressure)
- protection from radiation
- psoriasis and other skin problems
- raising HDL cholesterol (good cholesterol)

Can AKGs really support my immune system?

AKGs are noted to boost the immune system, even though it is not completely understood how it works. AKGs are instrumental in production and stimulation of white blood cells in bone marrow. Besides, Shark Liver Oil, AKGs are found in saltwater & freshwater fish, cows, and sheep.

Mother's milk has 10-times more AKG's than cow's milk. Your liver, spleen and bone marrow (part of the immune system), have AKGs. However, the most AKGs are found in deep water sharks!

Where can I get these AKGs?

AKGs are just one component of Shark Liver Oil. An authentic Shark Liver Oil product can be acquired from companies listed below at the end of this Special Report.

What about the other ingredient in Shark Liver Oil, Omega-3 oils?

Heart-health experts have found the benefits of eating fish are even greater than previously realized. In 1985 the New England Journal of Medicine found that *"the consumption of as little as one or two fish dishes per week may be of preventive importance in relation to coronary heart disease."* Omega-3 fats in fish benefits the heart by making the blood less prone to the abnormal clotting process that can lead to a heart attack.

Fresh fish rates high for keeping blood pressure in a healthy range. Jichi Medical School in Japan have shown that levels of *"good"* HDL cholesterol were high among Japanese who eat the most fish! Fish may also help those who suffer from arthritis.

According to Dr. Joel Kremer of Albany Medical College in New York, daily supplements of EPA (eicosapentaenoic acid) fish oil brought dramatic relief to inflammation and stiff joints caused by rheumatoid arthritis.

According to researchers at the University of Cincinnati, Ohio, researchers have successfully blocked both migraine headaches and kidney disease with Omega-3 fish oils. Migraines generally eased up in about 60 percent of those who took fish oil capsules for six weeks. The number of migraine attacks dropped from 2 per week to 02 every 02 weeks and they were less severe!

Those patients diagnosed early of kidney disease, showed a retardation of kidney deterioration by switching from animal fat to Omega-3 fish oils. According to Dr. Uno Barcelli, assistant professor of medicine at the University of Cincinnati, *"It seems fish oil must be used relatively early in the disease process."* Fish oil therapy had no effect on patients with advanced kidney disease. Remember, to acquire an authentic Shark Liver Oil supplement, please do your own research and ask folks at your local healthfood store.

"Natural Healing Benefits of Olive Oil!"

Olive oil varies in quality. The term *"virgin"* is loosely applied. Originally it meant that the oil was from the first pressing of the fruit, as opposed to the second or third pressing. Olive oil when unrefined has a greenish tinge and a pungent flavor. It is preferred to refined oils because the health qualities are intact.

Olive oil may be one of the best choices when cooking with oils. Olive oil IS NOT saturated fat but is a monounsaturated fatty acid, which is stable at high temperatures and less prone to oxidation than other vegetable oils. Extra Virgin Oil is probably your best choice of all the other oils.

People in the Mediterranean have been noted to develop far less heart disease than Americans, even though they drink, smoke and even consumed as much or more saturated fat than Americans! What are they doing different? Their diet consists of an oil they use on their vegetables, grain-rich dishes and meats. They even dip their bread in it! It's olive oil!

Yes, olive oil. One added bonus of monounsaturated fats, they maintain HDL (high density lipoprotein) that helps prevent heart disease. Olive, peanut and canola oils are noted to be highest in monounsaturated fats.

Insure you read the Nutrition Facts label on any cooking oil. Look for the word *"monounsaturated."* Look for the least amount of saturated fats and the most monounsaturated fats.

WARNING: INSURE you use *"cold pressed"* olive oil - Extra Virgin Olive Oil! Use all cooking oils sparingly!

Why are people who live by the Mediterranean Diet, healthier than Americans despite their high tobacco consumption, low exercise level and modest health-care system?

The Mediterranean Diet is a diet low in meat, but high in cereal, fruit, grain, legumes, monounsaturated fats-nuts and vegetables. Recent French Study found that the Mediterranean Diet after a heart attack was 70 percent more life-saving than the Standard American Diet (low-fat diet-less than 30 percent fat calories). Some Harvard Researchers favor the Mediterranean Diet over the Standard American Diet.

A research effort called the Seven Countries Study, examined 12,763 men ages 40 through 59 in the Netherlands, Finland, Italy, Greece, Croatia and Serbia, Japan and the United States.

Ten years after their initial screening, the study reported several important results:

- Mediterranean groups had lower death rates from all causes than the northern European and American groups.

- Lower mortality from coronary heart disease in Mediterranean countries.

- Men at the peak of their lives (45 years) have longer life expectancies in Greece than in any other European or North American country despite their high tobacco consumption, low exercise level and modest health-care system.

The Mediterranean Diet is based on traditional eating patterns evolving over centuries in Greece, Italy, North Africa, Southern France, Spain and several Middle Eastern nations. All share a general pattern of cooking and ingredients. The diet is rich in fruits, vegetables, legumes and grains.

The principal fat is olive oil! Lean red meat is eaten only a few times a month and in small portions. Eating foods from animal sources - namely dairy products, fish and poultry is low to moderate. Wine is drunk with meals. Plenty of crusty country-style bread is enjoyed with each meal.

The major fat used in the Mediterranean Diet is olive oil! Olive oil is primarily a monounsaturated fat, which is noted to lower harmful low-density lipoprotein (LDL) blood cholesterol and may increase good high-density lipoprotein (HDL) blood cholesterol. Olive oil isn't the only key to a healthy diet.
Here are some Mediterranean eating tips:

- Switch to olive oil (extra virgin).

- Avoid butter and margarine. There is nothing wrong with putting olive oil on toast or whole grain bread.

- Cut meat consumption. If you do eat meat, insure it's lean. Try small portions of poultry or fish with plenty of vegetables.

- INCREASE fruit and vegetable consumption.

- Eat plenty of whole grain bread. The darker the better (ingredients not burnt).

- Eat a salad at the beginning and end of each meal.

- Wine at each dinner meal. It's been noted that a couple glasses of wine each day may protect against coronary heart disease.

What is the BEST and Healthiest Olive Oil?

According to AARP Bulletin (April 2020), not all Olive Oil products are of the highest of qualities.

According to AARP Bulletin, look for the following 05 Points when you purchase Olive Oil:

- **1st Point:** Olive Oil should be Extra Virgin
- **2nd Point:** Olive Oil should be in a Dark Bottle or Tin (protect ingredients from direct light)
- **3rd Point:** Olive Oil should have 'Best-Before-Date.' Get an Olive Oil farthest from the 'Best-Before-Date.'
- **4th Point:** Olive Oil from California, USA. (Adheres to Standardized Testing).
- **5th Point:** Olive Oil Taste Test (slight burn in back of throat, has the highest levels of oleocanthal, a polyphenol that breaks-up Alzheimer's plaques).

Also, according to AARP Bulletin, cooking with Olive Oil gives off the least amounts of carcinogens (cancer causing compounds). Researchers heated various cooking oils to 437-degrees Fahrenheit, Olive Oil put out the least amounts of toxic compounds called alkenals.

"You Gotta Have Your Omega-3 Fatty Acids For Lunch And Dinner!"

Omega-3 Fatty Acids are made up of two components DHA & EPA! DHA which stands for docosahexaenoic acid. EPA stands for eicosapentaenoic acid. These two nutrients found in Omega-3 are noted to protect against heart disease, stroke, depression...

It was once thought that shellfish were hazardous to your cardiovascular system because they elevated blood cholesterol. Well it is just the opposite. Shellfish help protect arteries and blood vessels by significantly lowering bad-type blood cholesterol (LDL).

Shellfish carry high concentrations of Omega-3 fatty acids that help prevent blood clots (thrombi) in blood vessels and are noted to be potentially beneficial to many diseases to include allergies, asthma, cancer, headaches, psoriasis and rheumatoid arthritis!

Heart-health experts have found the benefits of eating fish are even greater than previously realized. In 1985 the New England Journal of Medicine found that *"the consumption of as little as one or two fish dishes per week may be of preventive importance in relation to coronary heart disease."*

Omega-3 fats in fish benefits the heart by making the blood less prone to the abnormal clotting process that can lead to a heart attack.

Fresh fish rates high for keeping blood pressure in a healthy range. Jichi Medical School in Japan have shown that levels of *"good"* HDL cholesterol were high among Japanese who eat the most fish! Fish may also help those who suffer from arthritis.

According to Dr. Joel Kremer of Albany Medical College in New York, daily supplements of EPA (eicosapentaenoic acid) fish oil brought dramatic relief to inflammation and stiff joints caused by rheumatoid arthritis.

Fish is less fattening and more digestible than beef. Fish is high in mineral selenium which has proven to chase away the blues. There are about twenty varieties of fish that can be purchased at your local supermarket.

Four ounces of fish furnishes anywhere from 89 calories to 236 calories, with raw haddock having the lowest calorie count of 89 and four ounces of canned herring rates the highest calorie count of 236.

- Salmon is low in saturated fat and high in Omega-3 fatty acids. Salmon provides only 233 calories per 4.5 ounce steak and only 06 grams of fat per 3 ounces.

According to researchers at the University of Cincinnati, Ohio, researchers have successfully blocked both migraine headaches and kidney disease with Omega-3 fish oils.

Migraines generally eased up in about 60 percent of those who took fish oil capsules for six weeks. The number of migraine attacks dropped from 02 per week to 02 every 02 weeks and they were less severe!

Those patients diagnosed early of kidney disease, showed a retardation of kidney deterioration by switching from animal fat to Omega-3 fish oils. According to Dr. Uno Barcelli, assistant professor of medicine at the University of Cincinnati, *"It seems fish oil must be used relatively early in the disease process."* Fish oil therapy had no effect on patients with advanced kidney disease.

English Nuts are five times more rich in Omega-3 fatty acids than all other nuts. Very few plant foods have this much Omega-3 fatty acids. English Nuts are also high in antioxidant anticancer allagic acid.

DHA an important essential fatty acid (Omega-3), is a major building block in gray matter of your brain. It also a major building block of the retina of your eye.

According to American Journal of Clinical Nutrition, *"Societies consuming large amounts of fish and Omega-3 fatty acids appear to have lower rates of major depression."*

WARNING: Fast food fish is noted to have 1/10 of Omega-3 fish oil compared to a can of Chinook salmon. Fast food fish is mostly made from whitefish already low in fat and Omega-3's.

Too much Omega-3 may block normal blood clotting and lead to excessive bleeding. Researchers have discovered that Omega-3 fish oil capsules can actually aggravate diabetes by producing a steep rise in blood sugar and a drop in insulin secretion.

"Amazing Healing Castor Oil!"

Can you give me some general information about Castor Oil?

Castor Oil is extracted from the castor bean plant and it's been used for thousands of years for just about every malady - sickness you can think of!

Castor Oil packs (more on this later) have been used with amazing results that most medical doctors would say is impossible. It is even taken internally.

Ask your own physician about the healing qualities and successes of Castor Oil. He\she may probably just laugh or discredit you and tell you to stay away from that nonsense! You have the right to investigate any alternative care practice - at least look into it.

Many varieties of sickly and deadly maladies have responded positively to the amazing healing qualities of Castor Oil. Castor Oil is a POTENT CLEANSER - DETOXIFIER! This means it gives your cleansed body the extra help the inherent ability to heal itself!

What is Castor Oil composed of?

Castor Oil is mainly composed of ricinoleic acid. Ricinoleic acid is an unsaturated hydroxy fatty acid. A high viscosity oil, some have described it as a nutritious oil.

It's noted to be an excellent emollient and lubricant as well as demonstrating antimicrobial activities. Below is a composition of Castor Oil:

- Ricinoleic acid--------------------89.5%
- Oleic acid------------------------03.0%
- Palmitic acid---------------------01.0%
- Stearic acid----------------------01.0%
- Dihydroxystearic acid-------------00.7%
- Eicosanoic acid-------------------00.3%
- Linoleic acid---------------------00.3%
- Linolenic acid--------------------00.3%

What is the healing secret to Castor Oil?
First of all, like many natural and extremely safe supplements like herbs, foods (raw fresh fruits & vegetables), miracle waters, other oils..., and 60 remarkable alternative healing therapies & treatments, research needs to be conducted! Research results you may NEVER see! Not in your lifetime.

Why many natural supplements and alternative therapies work - exactly work is unknown! There is a lot of good scientific evidence why many supplements work and why some Alternative Therapies work. But to find the EXACT reason why they any healing takes place needs much more research.

Heck, scientist and researchers are still conducting research on water - plain ol' water! I forget the name of the field of studying water - but that's all these scientists and researchers do - study water! And they'll be doing it as long as there is money to finance the research!

To come up with bonafide reasons why Castor Oil works along with hundreds of other alternative supplements and treatments & therapies - well don't hold your breath.

My best advice is to try to go back to the basics which is to use common sense and do what your doctor advises (as long as it works) and ALWAYS keep an open mind to other Alternatives Therapies that are safe and help your body to heal itself!

What are some healing benefits of Castor Oil?
The following is a partial list of reported healing results using Castor Oil packs. For many of the maladies listed below, a Castor Oil Pack on the abdomen has demonstrated remarkable results. Later you'll see how to make these healing Castor Oil packs.

- abdominal problems
- aching feet
- acne
- appendicitis

- arthritis
- back pain
- bath pruitis (itching)
- beautiful complexion
- cancer
- colitis
- constipation
- corns
- cyst
- ear problems
- edema of the ankles
- esophagus
- flactuence
- gall bladder conditions
- hearing loss
- hematoma (bleeding under the skin)
- hernias
- Hodgkin's Disease
- hyperactivity (tranquilizing effect)*
- inflammations
- liver conditions
- insomnia
- irregular-painful toe nails
- lesion
- liver spots
- migraine headaches
- Multiple Sclerosis
- nausea - vomiting
- pain

- Parkinson's Disease
- Ringworm
- sciatic pain
- severe skin abrasions (sans scars)
- skin abrasions
- skin cancer
- skin rash
- smashed or crushed finger - toe nails
- snoring (Castor Oil pack placed on abdomen)
- sprained ankle
- stretch marks
- vaginitis
- varicose veins
- warts

* Castor Oil pack on the belly.

How do I make Castor Oil Packs?

First of all, INSURE you have the cooperation and support of your doctor when using Castor Oil. Also insure you read additional and revealing information on Castor Oil (see below).

Below is a step-by-step list for making Castor Oil Packs:

a) Gather the following items:
   01) Bath Towel (white)
   02) Castor Oil (see Point of Contact)
   03) Clear plastic sheet
   04) Electric heating pad

05) Flannel cloth - large (wool)
06) Pan (10 x 14 inches)
06) Safety pins

b) Take you flannel cloth and fold it so that it is 02 to 04 layers and measures 10 by 14 inches. I'll give you a POC that offers Castor Oil as well as reusable wool flannel (18 X 24-abdominal & 12 X 18-other areas). Place the flannel cloth in the pan.

c) Pour Castor Oil in the pan and completely saturate the entire wool flannel cloth.

d) Remove the flannel and remove excess Castor Oil by wringing it out in the pan - but the it must be wet but not dripping wet.

e) Apply the saturated flannel cloth to the abdomen (stimulates the thymus - immune system for overall health) or the treated area.

f) Place a clear plastic sheet over the treated area followed by the heating pad. Set the heating pad on low and make adjustments if necessary.

g) Wrap the affected area with the white towel.

h) Castor Oil pack remains in place for 60 to 90 minutes and repeated daily - 03 to 07 days a week.

i) A plastic sheet may be placed on the bed if pack is used while laying down or sleeping.

j) Castor Oil packs may be reused as long as the oil doesn't become rancid. You can place them in clear plastic bags and place them in your refrigerator.

For other areas when using Castor Oil for external use, use smaller flannel pieces. You may also use gauze pads and even band-aids.

If you have aching feet, saturate a pair of white socks in Castor Oil and wear some old shoes or slippers while walking around or when sleeping!

Again, many times Castor Oil packs are placed on the abdomen which gets the immune system to *"kick-in"* its healing power! For other treated areas, simply apply the Castor Oil pack directly over the treated area.

Can I take Castor Oil internally?
Yes you can. I advise you to read any available materials on Castor Oil and I HIGHLY ADVISE you to seek advice from your physician.

What kind of Castor Oil should I get and where can I buy it?

Like Olive Oil, INSURE the Castor Oil you do by is:

a) Cold Pressed

b) Cold Processed

c) NO additives

Listed below are some Points Of Contact you should be aware of.

Association for Research
Enlightenment, Inc. (ARE)----------1-800-333-4499
                                  1-804-428-3588
                                  1-804-422-4631(fax)

Association for Research Enlightenment, Inc., (ARE) continues the work of a man named Edgar Cayce who founded the ARE in 1931. ARE is an international network of people and volunteers who are interested ancient civilizations, dream interpretation, ESP & psychic development, holistic healing, meditation, reincarnation, spiritual growth, the purpose of life, and much more.

There are many benefits to ARE members such as: ARE Camp, ARE Conferences and Seminars, ARE books by mail, The New Millennium Journal, Venture Inward Magazine, and much more. They'll send you a catalog of their books. One of which is called The Oil That Heals (Castor Oil). Call Monday through Friday from 8:00 a.m. to 5:00 p.m., Eastern Standard Time, for your free information packet!

"Super Healthy Flaxseed Oil!"

You've already read about the amazing healthy possibilities of Shark Liver Oil, Olive Oil, and Omega-3 Fatty Acids. Now let's talk about one more healthy oil you have to know about - Flaxseed Oil!

In 1909, the average U.S. person consumed approximately 125 grams of fat per day. Today the average person in the U.S. consumes approximately 175 grams of fat, an increase of 40 percent or about 50 extra pounds per year and increasing! Of the total increase in the consumption of fats and oils, shortening, margarine, refined salad oil and cooking oils account for fifty percent. This increase in fat over the years is undoubtedly linked to the increase in degenerative diseases.

In order to extend the shelf life of many products, essential fatty acids (good fat) have been purposely processed out of most foods. This is profitable for the manufacturer, but UNHEALTHY to the American consumer - YOU!

Approximately 80% of Americans are deficient in essential fatty acids. Flax seed has a high content of essential fatty acids.

Flax seed supplies the body with needed essential fatty acids and richer in Omega-3's than fish oil and packs more fiber ounce for ounce than oat bran!

Listed below are some observed benefits of flax seed:

- Seriously ill cancer patients were treated with flax seed oil and low-fat cottage cheese by Dr. Johanna Budwig. Over a period of approximately 90 days, tumors gradually receded. Symptoms of anemia, cancer, diabetes and liver dysfunction were completely alleviated!

- According to a study in Great Britain by Dr. Sinclair, a relative **deficiency of the essential fatty acids plays an important part in the causes** of arteriosclerosis, coronary thrombosis, diabetes mellitus, hypertension, multiple sclerosis and certain forms of malignant diseases!

- Dr. J.R. Vane shared the 1982 Nobel Prize for Medicine for his work proving how the metabolism of Omega-3 fatty acids helped prevent heart problems.

- A U.S. physician, Dr. Donald Rudin discovered that Omega-3 fatty acid deficiency is the basic cause of major mental illness, because fatty acids provide the substance upon which niacin and other B Vitamins act to form the prostaglandin-3 series tissue hormones which are special mission fatty acids that regulate neurocircuits through the whole body.

The Food and Drug Administration (FDA) has recently entered into a 03-year, $2 million contract with the National Cancer Institute (NCI) to research the effect of flax seed on various health concerns. The FDA will conduct experiments confirming flaxseed's role in fat and cholesterol metabolism, bone mineralization and the immune system. This research will make flaxseed one of the most intensively-studied nutrients used in any food product.

Flax seeds are a great source of healthy soluble and insoluble fiber as well as protein. Just 1/4 cup (50 grams) of flax seed provides 20 grams of fiber. Remember fiber is noted to ameliorate, heal, prevent:

- Colon cancer.
- Constipation.
- Diverticulosis.
- Hemorrhoids.
- Improves blood sugar metabolism.
- Lowers blood pressure.
- Lowers cholesterol.
- Protects against other cancers.
- Rectal cancer.
- Weight loss.
- Much more...

Follow the recommended dosage and instructions from the label and as per your doctor's instructions.

Now let's carry-on with *"Super Fighting & Healing Oil Of Oregano!"*

"Super Fighting & Healing Oil Of Oregano!"

Once you read this Special Report, I bet you're going to be so motivated to get this super healing wonder in your anxious hands, that you'll call the POC I'm going to give you within 10-seconds after you finish reading this very important Special Report.

This healthy data was taken directly from the 2005 Anytime Anywhere Survival Newsletter (2005 AASN) and is written in a Question and Answer format so you can better understand how powerful and important this healing wonder may be to you and your family member's benefit for the rest of your lives Anytime Anywhere! Are you ready? OK, let's get started with the history of healing oregano.

01) What is oregano and what is its healing history?
There are 60+ various species of oregano that come from the mint family, but very few oregano species have the super healing qualities we'll talk about in this Special Report. Oregano is commonly known as a seasoning herb, marjoram - (Origanum vulgare).

The antiseptic powers of oil of oregano are gigantic and make most other natural remedies and even synthetic drugs look weakly by comparison. Oil of oregano's wide and long resume of healings throughout history to the present day are very impressive (keep reading).

Without any assistance from other natural remedies or synthetic drugs, oregano kills fungus or blocks its growth. Oil of oregano also attacks and outright destroys antibiotic-resistant super-germs, bacteria, molds, parasites, viruses, yeast,...

In ancient times, the Greek Empire grew oregano along their hillsides. The Greeks used oregano for a variety of medicines which may explain why the Greeks were so powerful both mentally and physically.

Greek physicians used oregano to treat asthma, congestive heart failure, headaches, lung disorders, narcotic poisoning, open wounds, plant poisoning, seizures, venomous bites,... Approximately 3000 B.C., the Babylonians used oregano as a cure for lung and heart diseases. They also used oregano for treating wounds and venomous bites.

In the Middle Ages (476 AD to 1453 AD), Islamic physicians used oregano spices and oil of oregano as a germ killer. In the 9th century, a historian recorded that open markets in Baghdad, Iraq, sprinkled oregano on produce to keep it fresh. He recorded the vegetables went unspoiled for up to 02-weeks in the open air without any refrigeration.

Over thousands of years, oregano was eaten as food in the Mediterranean, Middle East, & Eastern Europe and each culture had their own oregano recipes. Some sprinkled oregano on their food while others added food to their oregano.

02) What types of healing oreganos are there?

There are oil of oregano, oregano juice and crushed wild oregano. The crushed wild oregano, the entire herb in its natural state is processed by being sun-dried. Oregano juice is the water soluble extract of wild oregano and processed and extracted by steam distillation. Oil of oregano is also produced by steam distillation.

True healing oregano grows wild on rock or calcium-loaded soils. Oregano is loaded with minerals like boron, calcium, copper, iron, magnesium, manganese, phosphorus, potassium, zinc,... Ounce for ounce amazing super oregano has 16-times more calcium than milk. And its heavily loaded with zinc, ounce for ounce, more zinc than cheese, peanut butter, salmon, sardines,... Oregano also contains Vitamins like beta carotene, niacin, riboflavin (B complex), thiamine (B complex), Vitamin C, and Vitamin K. And oregano has anti-oxidant qualities, fighting free-radicals that cause disease, aging,... Oregano could be considered a super food.

03) What are the healing ingredients in oregano?

Oil of oregano contains a host of ingredients to carvacrol - its main ingredient. Carvacrol is a phenol which is a powerful antiseptic. It also contains another phenol called thymol. Together both phenols work synergistically, meaning the combination is more powerful together than alone.

Oil of oregano contains more than 50 compounds that possess antimicrobial functions with carvacrol and thymol being the main ingredients. Other ingredients include: Alpha-humulene, Amyl Furan, Beta-Bisabolene, Beta-Caryophyllene, Camphene, Carene, Cineole, Cis-dihydrocarvone, Cis-sabinene Hydrate, Cymene, Decane, Germacrene D, Hexanal, Hexenal, Limonene, Linalool, Linalyl Acetate, Methyl Carvacrol, Myrcene, Nonanal, Nonane, Ocimene, Phellandrene, Pinene, Sabinene, Spathcoulane, Terpinen-4-ol, Terpinene, Terpinolene, Thymol, Trans-dihydrocarvone, Undecane,...

A study at Georgetown University Medical Center, Washington D.C., headed by Harry G. Preuss, M.D., tested the efficacy of oregano against Candida albicans (yeast infection) and found that oregano *"can act as a potent antifungal agent against Candida albicans."* Business Weekly magazine states *"Oregano could turn into the next wonder drug."*

04) Go back to the fungus part. Fungus is dangerous isn't it?
It surely is. Fungus lives off dead or dying tissue and it lives among live tissue outside and inside your body that causes all types of sickly maladies.

Listen to this, health-care in the United States runs more than a trillion dollars a year! Yet Americans are the most chronically sickliest people on Earth. More than 60% of all Americans are overweight.

And Americans are the most fungally infested people on Earth and fungus is responsible for a many sickly maladies, some of which eventually leading to a costly sickly death.

Here's a good reason why Americans are the most fungally infested people on Earth. American love sugar, Americans are addicted to sugar. Just about every food, drink, and snack that is consumed by Americans has sugar in it.

On the average, each American consumes a whopping 150-pounds of sugar each year! That's about 06 1/2-ounces of sugar each day! And that sugar is a food source for fungus, fungus that's inside you right now. No wonder you feel or are sick all the time.

And fungi are a survivor, it's difficult to kill. In nuclear bomb testing of the 1940s and 1950s, microbes were tested against radiation fallout. It turned out that Candida albicans, a fungus\yeast, survived the deadly fallout. Fungi is a survivor, difficult to kill, yet oil of oregano attacks and kills fungi easily, it's no contest.

And as I stated earlier, oil of oregano also attacks and outright destroys antibiotic-resistant super-germs, bacteria, molds, parasites, viruses, yeast,...

05) Why haven't I heard about super healing oregano before now?

The true healing oregano products haven't been around that long. They were introduced in the United States about 1996. At the same time there are federal laws prohibiting *"cure-all"* advertising. Plus, when folks do read the amazing super healing testimonials of oregano, most think it's too good to be true.

06) Are these super healing oregano products a cure-all?

It sure seems like they are but they're not, no one natural or man-made medicine is a cure-all. These super healing oregano products help your body to heal itself by going after the antibiotic-resistant super-germs, bacteria, fungus, molds, parasites, viruses, yeast,... inside and outside your body so your immune system can fight better to heal you.

With super healing oregano products, your immune system is no longer out-manned and out-gunned by antibiotic-resistant super-germs, bacteria, fungus molds, parasites, viruses, yeast,... invading your body.

07) What are some noted benefits of super healing oregano products?

Here's an exceptionally long list of what oregano kills (bad guys), as well as its benefits for ameliorating a wide variety of disorders. And this isn't a complete listing either.

Odds are YOU or someone close to you is troubled by one or more of the following health maladies and should take a closer look at super healing oil of oregano. OK, here's that list in alphabetical order:

Note: As I've always said *"Try the least intrusive method(s) first to remedy your health problem before going forward with conventional medicine of drugs and/or surgery."*

- Acne
- Alcoholic Neuritis
- Allergies
- Animal Bites
- Arthritis
- Asthma
- Athlete's Foot
- Back Pain
- Bad Breath
- Bed Sores
- Bladder Infections
- Boils
- Bromidrosis (body odor)
- Bronchitis
- Bruises
- Burns
- Bursitis
- Candidiasis
- Canker Sores
- Cellulitis
- Chicken Pox

- Cholera
- Colds
- Cold Sores
- Colitis
- Congestion
- Constipation
- Cough
- Crohn's Disease
- Croup
- Dandruff
- Dengue Fever
- Dental Cavities
- Dermatitis
- Diaper Rash
- Diarrhea
- Diphtheria
- Diverticulitis
- Ear Aches
- Ear Infections
- Ebola
- Eczema
- Emphysema
- Encephalitis (includes West Nile virus)
- Esophagitis
- Fatigue
- Fingernail Fungus
- Flactuence
- Flu
- Food Poisoning

- Frostbite
- Frostburn
- Gastritis
- Genital Herpes
- Giardiasis
- Gonorrhea
- Gout
- Gum Disease
- Hantavirus
- Headaches
- Hepatitis
- Hiatal Hernia
- Hives
- Impetigo (skin infection)
- Ingrown Toenail
- Insect Bites
- Irritable Bowel Syndrome
- Jock Itch
- Kidney Infection
- Kills Amebas
- Kills Antibiotic-Resistant Super-Germs
- Kills Bacteria
- Kills Camphylobacter
- Kills Clostridium
- Kills Cryptosporidium
- Kills Cyclospora
- Kills E. Coli
- Kills Enterobacter

- Kills Fleas
- Kills Flukes Cholera
- Kills Fungus
- Kills Germs
- Kills Giardia
- Kills Lice
- Kills Parasites
- Kills Salmonella
- Kills Shigella
- Kills Viruses
- Kills Worms
- Kills Yeast
- Laryngitis
- Leaky Gut Syndrome
- Leg Cramps
- Listeria
- Low Blood Pressure
- Lower Lung Conditions
- Lyme Disease
- Malaria
- Measles
- Mumps
- Nail Fungus
- Neuritis
- Open Wounds
- Oral Lesions
- Paronychia (nail infection)
- Peptic Ulcer
- Pneumatic Conditions

- Pneumonia
- Poison Ivy
- Poison Oak
- Poison Sumac
- Psoriasis
- Prostate Disorders
- Prostatis
- Pruritus (itchy skin)
- Radiation Injuries
- Rash
- Ring Worm
- Rosacea (face rash)
- Scabies
- Seborrhea
- Shingles
- Sinusitis
- Skin Cancer
- Sleeping Sickness
- Sore Throat
- Spider Bites
- Spinal Infection
- Splinters
- Sports Injuries
- Stomach Disorders
- Sunburn
- Tartar
- Tendinitis
- Thrush (mouth infection)
- Tick-borne Illness

- Tooth Abscess
- Toothache
- Tonsillitis
- Tuberculosis
- Upper Respiratory Tract Conditions
- Urinary Infection
- Varicose Veins
- Venomous Bites
- Vitiligo (skin pigment)
- Warts
- Wounds
- AND MORE...

08) How do I know how to use oregano for a particular malady?

First, so I won't get sued by some weasel money-hungry lawyer, I have to tell you that this Special Report like everything else in this IRISAP Survival Program is for *"informational use only."* Second, you must see your physician before you engage in any alternative supplement.

Odds are your doctor might say *"baaa hum bug"* and prescribe more drugs. However, YOU and YOU ALONE are the final approving authority for your precious health. Without your health, you got diddly squat - no matter how rich you are.

OK, now to answer your question. I'm way ahead of you, below is a GREAT book you have to get for valuable information on super healing oregano. This 203-page book will give you all the information you need to act upon for this super healing herb.

Plus, when you send for FREE information from the POC below, they also give doses and instructions for their authentic oregano products.

09) Are there fake oregano products out there?

Yes, you bet there are. Not until 1996 were true medicinal oregano products available in the United States. Before this time and the present, fake oregano products appear on healthfood store shelves throughout the country. These fake oregano products have little or no medicinal qualities. Fake oregano products that carry the name but are products like marjoram oil, Spanish oregano, thyme oil,...

10) Where can I read more about super healing oregano?

Here is a book you have to get as soon as possible (beg borrow or go to your local library):

The Cure Is In The Cupboard-------by Dr. Cass Ingram
(How To Use Oregano For Better Health). I used this book as one of my references for this Special Report.

"STOP Toothache Pain With This Super Oil!"

Folks, I want to make sure you get your money's worth, so here's another late entry. This is going to be very brief but extremely worthy of your attention when no dentist is available for a really bad toothache pain.

In late July of 2013, I was suffering from a non-stop toothache pain from hell. I swished and gargled with salt water which actually helped out a bit but the pain came back. I dental flossed repeatedly trying to remove any debris that may have been caught between the tooth and gum and I massaged the area practically non-stop trying to get more blood in the area. But the horrible toothache pain miserably occupied my life every second for about 02-days.

I gotta tell you, they could throw that water-boarding interrogation technique (Chinese Water Torture) out the window and give that prisoner a plain ol' fashion killer toothache from hell and that prisoner will soon start talking non-stop and beg for a dentist to relieve his awful pain.

As always, I conducted some *"intensive research"* to solve my aching problem. Finally, I think I found the healing answer to my toothache pain without spending several hundred dollars for an emergency dentist visit.

But to make sure I keyed on this healing oil and conducted more research or was it too occupy myself so to try to get my mind off the nagging toothache pain.

Well, I decided this oil was going to be my healer, my banishment for this cussing toothache pain from hell. I got in my car and ended up driving at least 02-hours trying to this elusive oil. I tried GNC - they were out of it. I tried another GNC, they were closed. I tried Walgreen - what kind of oil did you say? I finally found a Mom & Pop health food store and they had it!!!

I purchased it and walked out the door and went to another store to buy some cotton balls and some Q-Tips. Returning to my car, I applied this Special Oil right in the parking lot.

OK, OK, what kind of oil are you talking about?

This special oil is called Clove Oil (*Eugenia caryophyllata*) {Ingredients: 100% pure clove oil}. The 01-fluid ounce (30 mL) dark bottle cost $6.99 plus taxes. Here's a step-by-step process of what I did to STOP my toothache in less than 02-minutes.

Step 01: Apply 03 or 04 drops of Clove Oil to a single Q-Tip.

Step 02: Massage the treated Q-Tip to the tooth or teeth for 15-seconds.

STEP 03:   Massage the same treated Q-Tip to the surrounding gum area for 15-seconds.

Step 04:   Go ahead and spit, cause Clove Oil has a strong scented taste to it.

STEP 05:   Repeat Steps 01 thru 04.   You'll find after the 1st treatment the toothache pain is already diminishing.   At the end of the 2nd treatment, the toothache pain is completely gone – well this is what happened to me.   And the toothache pain never returned.

Clove Oil goes after the bad guys (germicide, bactericide,…), so I think I had a bad infection and the Clove Oil went after it.   Bottom line – it STOPPED my non-stop toothache pain within a couple minutes.   I hope you can use this info in the future when no dentist is immediately available.

OK, now let's carry-on with *Wheat Germ Oil For After Burner Performance*!

"Wheat Germ Oil For After-Burner Performance!"

Here's a health supplement worthy of your attention and it may give you that after-burner performance. This healthy supplement is called wheat germ oil. Wheat germ is part of the wheat plant that's responsible for sprouting and making new wheat plants.

The wheat germ is alive with life and is made-up of proteins, vitamins, and minerals. Just a half-cup of wheat germ contains 24 grams of protein. It includes minerals like calcium, copper, manganese, magnesium, and potassium. It also includes B Vitamins, and Vitamin E.

Now wheat germ oil is pressed out of the wheat germ. The wheat germ oil is rich in fat soluble Vitamins. According to Dr. T. K. Cureton, head of the University of Illinois Physical Fitness Laboratory, wheat germ oil may help maintain endurance in athletic performance.

A single daily teaspoon of wheat germ oil along with exercise has shown to increase men's physical endurance by as much as a whopping 51%! This amazing find was based on Dr. Cureton's 04-year research that includes tests on 200 men including college men, middle-aged men, swimmers, wrestlers,...

According to Dr. Cureton, *"Wheat germ oil is a valuable dietary supplement to men doing hard exercise, and it has possible application to competitive sports. We have tried it sufficiently to believe that this is true. It provides something that enables men to bear hard stress and continue to do hard labor without deteriorating. It particularly affects physical endurance and heart response."*

Note: All the B Vitamins aid to maintain healthy eyes, hair, liver, mouth, muscle tone in the gastrointestinal tract, nerves and skin. B-Complex Vitamins are coenzymes involved in energy production. B-Complex Vitamins may be useful to combat depression or anxiety. The B Vitamins should be taken together.

"Other Healthy Uses Of Wheat Germ!"

VITAMIN B1 (THIAMINE): Vitamin B1 enhances circulation and assists in the production of hydrochloric acid, blood formation, and carbohydrate formation. Vitamin B1 affects energy, growth disorders and learning capacity.

Vitamin B1 is needed for muscle tone of the intestines, stomach, and heart. Thiamin is noted as a brain booster because it helps produce the messages your brain sends out to nerve cells. Thiamin is vital to memory and learning.

Sources of Vitamin B1 are asparagus, broccoli, Brussels sprouts, dried beans, brown rice, egg yolks, fish, organ meats (kidney, liver, heart), many nuts, oatmeal, peanuts, peas, plums, pork, poultry, dried prunes, raisins, rice bran, sardines, soybeans, turkey, **wheat germ**, and whole grain.

Vitamin B1 is noted to repel bugs! Many testimonials of outdoors people have noted that mosquitoes simply want nothing to do with you. According to one study, Vitamin B1 did not prevent mosquito bites (controlled study) but may help in the prevention of the pain and itching brought on by the bites. Consuming sulfur, like garlic, is also noted to have repelling effect on many insects including mosquitoes.
Follow the recommended dosage and instructions from the label and as per your doctor's instructions.

VITAMIN B6 (PYRIDOXINE): According to the Food and Nutrition Board of the National Research Council, it has determined the Recommended Dietary Allowance of Vitamin B6 for adult males is 2mg and 1.6mg for adult females per day. <u>Vitamin B6 is involved in more bodily functions than any other nutrient. Vitamin B6 affects both physical and mental health</u>. Vitamin B6 is beneficial for those suffering from water retention.

This Vitamin is essential for the production of hydrochloric acid as well as the absorption of fats and protein.

This Vitamin aids in maintaining sodium and potassium balance while promoting red blood cell formation. Vitamin B6 is required by the nervous system, needed for normal brain function and synthesis of RNA and DNA. This Vitamin activates many enzymes and aids in B12 absorption, immune system function, and antibody production.

Vitamin B6 plays a role in cancer immunity and arteriosclerosis. This Vitamin inhibits the formation of a toxic chemical called homocysteine. Homocysteine attacks the heart muscle and allows the deposition of cholesterol around the heart muscle. Pyridoxine may also be useful in preventing oxalate kidney stones.

It also acts as a mild diuretic. Vitamin B6 (Pyridoxine) reduces symptoms of premenstrual syndrome. It also helps in the treatment of allergies, arthritis, and asthma. Carpal tunnel syndrome is linked to Pyridoxine deficiency. The lack of Vitamin B6 may enhance the formation of coronary artery blockages.

Sources of Vitamin B6 are from all foods. However, significant sources of Vitamin B6 are avocado, bananas, beans, brown rice, cabbage, cantaloupe, carrots, chicken, eggs, fish, meat, peas, spinach, sunflower seeds, walnuts, **wheat germ**, and whole grains.

WARNING: Antidepressants, estrogen, and oral contraceptives may increase the need for Vitamin B6 in the body. Extremely high doses of Vitamin B6 can be toxic.
Follow the recommended dosage and instructions from the label and as per your doctor's instructions.

VITAMIN E: According to the Food and Nutrition Board of the National Research Council, it has determined the Recommended Dietary Allowance of Vitamin E for adult males is 10mg per day and for adult females is 8mg per day. Vitamin E is an antioxidant that prevents cancer and cardiovascular disease!

Vitamin E improves circulation, repairs tissue, and is useful in treating fibrocystic breast and premenstrual syndrome. Vitamin E promotes normal clotting and healing, reduces scarring from wounds, reduces blood pressure, aids in preventing cataracts, improves athletic performance, and aids in leg cramps! Vitamin E prevents cell damage and the formation of free radicals as well as retards aging and may prevent age spots. Zinc is essential to maintain proper levels of Vitamin E in the blood.

Sources of Vitamin E are dry beans, brown rice, cornmeal, cold-pressed vegetable oils, eggs, desiccated liver, milk, oatmeal, organ meats, sweet potatoes, **wheat germ**, whole grains, dark green leafy vegetables, nuts, and seeds. Processing, storage, and cooking cause some loss of Vitamin E from foods.

Did you know there's a fruit-derived substance that has 20 times more antioxidant activity than Vitamin C and 50 times more antioxidant activity than Vitamin E? It's non-toxic and effective. It's called Oligometric Proanthocyanidin and it's called Grape Seed Phytosome and it's from Enzymatic Therapy.

WARNING: Do not take iron and Vitamin E at the same time. People suffering from diabetes, rheumatic heart disease, or an overactive thyroid should not use high doses. People suffering from high blood pressure should start with a small amount and increase slowly to the desired amount (Seek advice from your Doctor). Follow the recommended dosage and instructions from the label and as per your doctor's instructions.

IMPOTENCE: Impotence is an inability to maintain an erection of the penis. Causes of impotence are alcoholism, antidepressants, antihistamines, chemotherapy for cancer (generalized weakness), decreased hormonal levels, eating foods containing Diethylstilbestrol (causes destruction of virility in men), estrogen (treatment for prostate cancer), heating the genitals (by saunas or hot tubs), high blood pressure medications, hypothyroidism, hypogonadism, low blood sugar, lowered pineal gland and hippocampus function, narcotics (decreased libido), organic nervous conditions, overconsumption of caffeine, psychological nervous conditions, scar tissue from previous surgery in the gonadal area, smoking (constricts arteries in the gonadal area causing decreased blood supply), tranquilizers (decreases sex drive and causes nerve blockage), ulcer medications, and wearing tight pants (slows down the production of male hormones).

Oysters and clams are rich in zinc, an important mineral for prostate gland function, normal sperm count and sexual libido. Other sources of zinc are **wheat germ** and organ meats.

Folic Acid -- Folic acid is considered brain food and needed for energy production and formation of red blood cells. It helps with protein metabolism. In addition to protecting against adult diseases, folic acid reduces the risk of birth defects in a fetus's developing nervous system by 50 percent!

The evidence is so strong that the Centers for Disease Control and Prevention (CDC) recommends that all women who may become pregnant consume 400mcg of folic acid a day. Folic Acid helps regulate embryonic and fetal development of nerve cells, vital for normal growth and development. Folic Acid works best with Vitamin B12. A sore, red tongue may be one sign of Folic Acid deficiency.

Significant sources of Folic Acid are barley, beans, beef, bran, brown rice, cheese, chicken, dates, green leafy vegetables, lamb, lentils, liver, milk, oranges, organ meats, split peas, pork, root vegetables, tuna, **wheat germ**, whole grains, whole wheat and yeast.

WARNING: Oral contraceptives may increase the need for Folic Acid. High doses of Folic Acid for extended periods should be avoided by anyone with a hormone-related cancer or convulsive disorder.

WHEAT GERM WEIGHT-LOSS: Wheat germ is part of the wheat plant that's responsible for sprouting and making new wheat plants. The wheat germ is <u>alive with life</u> and is made-up of proteins, vitamins and minerals. Anyway, quite some time back, I interviewed a friend who told me their mother lost weight using wheat germ.

All she did was add wheat germ to EVERYTHING she ate. From breakfast to dinner meals and even snacks, wheat germ was always part of the meal. It was as simple as that. I use *Kretschmer Wheat Germ*. It's an excellent healthy food additive.

Note: Try a hefty combination of Wheat Germ (03 tablespoons), Sprouts (02 handfuls) and your favorite salad dressing for a super healthy meal.

"The Many Amazing Healings And Uses Of Coconut Oil!"

Here's some super healthy data on coconuts and why you should not only take fresh coconuts on all your outdoor adventures but also have coconut slices in your trail-mix. Instead of just focusing on coconut oil, I decided to give more heathy data on this amazing food and healer. Let's start talking about *Electrolytes*.

Electrolytes: According to Cookycoconuts.com, nutritional values change as the coconut matures. Move aside Gatorade - for the liquid inside the coconut is coconut water or called coconut juice and is one of the HIGHEST sources of electrolytes on Earth. Electrolytes are ionized salts in blood, tissue fluids and cells including salts of sodium and potassium. A substance that can conduct electricity when it is in solution. So? So what?

We need electrolytes because our entire body is an electrical system and we need those electrolytes to keep us performing at our best whether we're running in a marathon or sitting behind a desk.

Coconut Juice: The coconut juice (milk) is consumed to prevent dehydration and is used in some areas of the world to hydrate casualties via intravenous tubes and needles. See *Coconut Water*.

Coconut Oil: The fresh white coconut meat is protein rich and loaded with coconut oil. Coconut oil is rich in what is called lauric acid which is found in Mother's milk. Lauric acid has anti-bacteria, anti-fungal, and anti-viral agents. The super healthy fresh coconut oil and fresh white meat have a laundry list of super healthy benefits like:

- Anti-Bacteria
- Anti-Fungal
- Anti-Viral
- Candida Albicans
- Chronic Fatigue
- Chron's Disease
- Diabetes
- Digestive Disorders
- Energy Booster
- Heart Disease
- IBS (irritable bowel syndrome
- Immune System Booster
- Lowers Cholesterol
- Metabolism Booster
- Rejuvenate Skin
- Thyroid Function

- Weight-Loss
- Wrinkles

Bottom line, now you know plenty of good reasons to mix plenty of fresh coconut slices in your trial-mix.

Note: Cookycoconuts.com recommends the best brand coconut oil is Tropical Traditions.

Pacific Coconut Parts: Here are some coconut parts and their uses by Pacific Islanders. OK, let's start with coconut roots:

a) Roots: Roots were used to make medicine and used as a fertilizer.

b) Trunk: The trunk of the coconut tree is durable and hard wood to make furniture, used for many construction projects, used to make bridges (*Bridge Over The River Kwai?*).

c) Bark: The bark (towards the top of the tree) of the coconut tree is used to make strainers, rags, clothing, sandals,...

d) Blossom Sheath: The blossom sheath (tops of tree where young coconut nuts emerge) is used for firewood, used for funnels, toys,...

e) Blossom: The blossom is tapped for tuba. Tuba is a white coconut sap. Tuba can be prepared and used a few ways like a sweetener, alcoholic beverage, vinegar, or a syrup.

f) Nut Stems: The nut stems are used for decoration, firewood, fertilizer,...

g) Baby Nut: The young baby nut can be used for food, toys,...

h) Immature Nut: The young coconut nut's husk is used to make rope, to buff, wipe, sponge, toilet paper, fertilizer,... It's burned to produce a smudge to repel mosquitoes. It can be carved to make flatware,...

i) Young Shell: The young shell is young enough, can be eaten.

j) Mature Coconut: The hard shell can be carved to make various tools, weapons, flatware,... The 02 empty halves can be used as a bra. The hard shell is a great kindling.

k) Coconut Meat: The coconut meat is used to make a sauce, candy, soap, coconut oil,...

Note: Nowhere have I found evidence of coconut meat being used as kindling. - **www.survivalexpert.com/fire**

l) **Leaf:** The durable leaves are used for paddles, stirring utensil,...

m) **Ribs:** The ribs of the coconut leaves - namely the stems, are used to make toothpicks for dental hygiene, make brooms,...

n) **Fronds:** The thinner leaves of the coconut tree are called fronds and are used for weaving to make baskets, fans, hats, mats,...

o) **Milk:** The coconut milk is a very beneficial drink.

Coconut Water: Here are several benefits of Coconut Water.

a) **Coconut Water:** In this segment we'll concentrate on coconut water. Coconut water comes from the **young green coconuts** versus the coconut milk that comes from mature coconuts. Young fresh coconuts can be purchased from specialty healthfood stores. You may also put in a request for *"young green coconuts."*

b) **Coconut Water:** Coconut water helps lower bad cholesterol levels (HDL) that are a risk for heart disease. Coconut water also helps with digestion, improves libido, dissolves kidney stones, and fights bladder and urinary tract infections. An old Philippine saying goes something like *'A coconut a day keeps the urologist away.'*

c) Fluid of Life: Some natives around the world where coconuts are found, call the coconut the *"Fluid of Life."*

d) Hydration: If you're dehydrated whether in a survival situation, athletic sports or after a binge of drinking,... coconut water may be the quick remedy to quick hydration. Plus, you get the nutrition and electrolytes much needed by the dehydrated body.

Coconut water can be used to fight-off dehydration by drinking it prior, during and after forecasted events where the body is physically stressed.

e) Blood Replacement: The electrolytes found in coconut water are about the same levels found in your plasma. Electrolytes are ionized salts in blood, tissue fluids and cells including salts of sodium and potassium. A substance that can conduct electricity when it is in solution. So? So what? We need electrolytes because our entire body is an electrical system and we need those electrolytes to keep us performing at our best whether we're running in a marathon or sitting behind a desk. In emergency situations, coconut water can be used as a substitute for blood.

f) Nutritious: Coconut water provides calcium, chloride, magnesium, potassium,... while its low in protein, sodium, sugar,... Plus, like I said it's loaded with electrolytes.

g) Other Benefits Of Coconut Water: Researchers out of India found that coconut water may aid in reducing symptoms of heart disease. Different studies found that coconut water may help to detoxify the liver. And coconut water may aid to lower bad cholesterol (LDL).

h) PMS Cure: This segment comes from Woman's World Magazine, by Amy Capetta (13 February 2007 - [page 26). As a young lady, Katie developed all out PMS in her 20s!

Trying every remedy she knew, nothing worked and she was a sickly mess with severe mood swings, fatigue, headaches, cramps, irritable bowel syndrome,... Finally, a friend told her to try coconut water. Katie drank a 12-ounce bottle of coconut water 03-times a week. Noticing little changes almost immediately, it was only 03-weeks later she realized she wasn't stricken with severe mood swings, fatigue, headaches, cramps, irritable bowel syndrome,... Now she drinks coconut water BEFORE and DURING each period. Katie says: *"Thanks to coconut water, all my days are good."*

i) Genuine Coconut Water Products: Genuine Coconut Water can be purchased at some healthfood stores. Some name brands that offer a genuine coconut water are O.N.E., VitaCoco and Zico. Look for Coconut Water at your local healthfood store. Now let's carry-on with *NG Trobriand Skinny Diet*.

NG Trobriand Skinny Diet: Since most Americans are overweight, I thought I'd add this diet. In the South Pacific lay the Trobriand Islands and obesity is about non-existent. Why? They eat no fried foods. As a matter of fact, their diet is mainly composed of fish, coconuts, and steamed vegetables. It's that simple. (National Geographic - July 1992)

Bacteria Proof: The outer shell of the coconut (young and old) keeps bacteria and parasites away from the liquid and meat of the coconut.

Pacific Cavity Free Teeth: Yapese adults carry a betel-nut basket that is hand-woven. The betel-nut basket holds aged or hollow coconut shell that are filled with lime powder. The lime powder is made from crushed coral. The coconut shell also holds betel nuts and leaves. The betel nut is split open and sprinkled with lime powder. This is wrapped in a leaf and chewed. The betel nut releases a red dye which reddens - stains the teeth and gums and has been used for ages to make their teeth cavity-proof.

HOLD THE PHONE - HOLD THE PHONE!!!

Swishing Away Toothache Pain In Minutes: Several pages up, you already read - *"STOP Toothache Pain With This Super Oil!"*

For the last several years *Clove Oil* has 100% of the time cured any 'toothache PAIN from hell' I had – till now.

Today is Monday – 05 March 2018. The last several days I've had a toothache and have used Clove Oil. The Clove Oil worked but the toothache came back agaon and again. The last 02 nights the toothache kept me awake. This morning at 0230 hours (2:30am), I got up and had to do something. So I tried **Oil Pulling**. You'll read about *Oil Pulling* about 15 pages ahead. Go ahead and read that segment right now and come back here when you're done.

Anyway, I scraped some coconut oil (in a hard state depending on the temperature) with a spoon into a small pot and heated it up. I then transferred the liquid coconut oil into a measuring cup and poured it into my mouth.

Most experts will say swish around the coconut oil for 15 to 20 minutes. So I set the timer to 15-minutes cause I really didn't like standing around for 15-minutes swishing around coconut oil in my mouth. So the timer started and I was swishing the coconut oil around in my mouth and trying to swish it on the bottom right-side where the toothache pain was located. Every minute or so air would take-up space in my mouth from all the swishing so I pointed my mouth upward and let out the excess air and continued swishing.

Finally, the 15-minutes was up and I was REALLY FEELING LESS TOOTHACHE PAIN! So I reset the timer on the stove for 05 more minutes to do the full 20-minutes. After 20-minutes of swishing the coconut oil around in my mouth, I spit out the coconut oil in the trash container.

Again, I was REALLY FEELING LESS TOOTHACHE PAIN! So I went to bed, and now I'm up and there is NO NAGGING TOOTHACHE PAIN!! I'M A REAL BELIEVER NOW! I already believed *Oil Pulling* works, but now I'M A REAL BELIEVER. So in about 10 more minutes I'm going to do some more Oil Pulling for a full 20-minutes to INSURE that nagging toothache doesn't come back.

Coconut Points Of Contact:

Coconut Nutrition----------www.cookycoconuts.com

Tropical Traditions--------www.tropicaltraditions.com
Offers high quality virgin coconut oil that is not processed and tainted like most inferior coconut oils.

OK, now let's carry-on with an amazing oil called *Panaseeda*.

"Fish Oil – The Healing Facts!"

Fish And Fish Oil: Heart-health experts have found the benefits of eating fish are even greater than previously realized. In 1985 the New England Journal of Medicine found that *"the consumption of as little as one or two fish dishes per week may be of preventive importance in relation to coronary heart disease."* Omega-3 fats in fish benefits the heart by making the blood less prone to the abnormal clotting process that can lead to a heart attack.

Fresh fish rates high for keeping blood pressure in a healthy range. Jichi Medical School in Japan have shown that levels of *"good"* HDL cholesterol were high among Japanese who eat the most fish! Fish may also help those who suffer from arthritis.

According to Dr. Joel Kremer of Albany Medical College in New York, daily supplements of EPA (eicosapentaenoic acid) fish oil brought dramatic relief to inflammation and stiff joints caused by rheumatoid arthritis.

Fish is less fattening and more digestible than beef. Fish is high in mineral selenium which has proven to chase away the blues.

There are about twenty varieties of fish that can be purchased at your local supermarket. Four ounces of fish furnishes anywhere from 89 calories to 236 calories, with raw haddock having the lowest calorie count of 89 and four ounces of canned herring rates the highest calorie count of 236.

- Salmon is low in saturated fat and high in Omega-3 fatty acids. Salmon provides only 233 calories per 04.5 ounce steak and only 06 grams of fat per 03 ounces.

According to researchers at the University of Cincinnati, Ohio, they have successfully blocked both migraine headaches and kidney disease with Omega-3 fish oils.

Migraines generally eased up in about 60 percent of those who took fish oil capsules for six weeks. The number of migraine attacks dropped from 02 per week to 02 every 02 weeks and they were less severe!

Those patients diagnosed early with kidney disease, showed a retardation of kidney deterioration by switching from animal fat to Omega-3 fish oils.

According to Dr. Uno Barcelli, assistant professor of medicine at the University of Cincinnati, *"It seems fish oil must be used relatively early in the disease process."* Fish oil therapy had no effect on patients with advanced kidney disease.

Is fish a brain food? It sure is! Fish is noted to be food for thought! According to Dr. Judith Wurtman, principal investigator at MIT, the high protein in fish, namely the amino acid tyrosine, may boost the brain neurotransmitters norepinephrine and dopamine, which energizes your mind and makes you feel more alert. Three or four ounces of fish (broiled or grilled) is sufficient.

WARNING: Fast food fish is noted to have 1/10 of Omega-3 fish oil compared to a can of Chinook salmon. Fast food fish is mostly made from whitefish already low in fat and Omega-3's.

Too much Omega-3 may block normal blood clotting and lead to excessive bleeding. Researchers have discovered that Omega-3 fish oil capsules can actually aggravate diabetes by producing a steep rise in blood sugar and a drop in insulin secretion.

See *Krill Oil*.

"The Amazing Healings Of Panaseeda Oil!"

First let me tell you I'm not making a single penny for telling you about Panaseeda Oil.

The reason I added Panaseeda Oil to this Survival Book is because of the story I read about a German - a 1996 Olympian named Andreas Wecker who won a Gold Medal on the High Bar and won other Olympic Medals. An athlete in phenomenal shape who years later (early 2000s), his health declined in the worst way.

In 2005 his health declined so much he weighed-in at a sickly 84 pounds. Andreas Wecker was diagnosed with chronic sickness called Crohn's disease (inflammatory bowel disease). Close to death, Andreas Wecker turned to an alternative treatment where every conventional method failed.

Below is a website where you can get the whole detailed story.

Get on the internet and typed the following into the search bar:

Andreas Wecker - Panaseeda Oil

Several websites should come up. You decide if Panaseeda Oil is a healthy option for you. See your doctor for professional medical advice.

"Healing Tea Tree Oil From Down Under!"

What is Tea Tree Oil?
Tea Tree Oil also called Melaleuca oil and is taken from the leaves of the small tree or shrub called Melaleuca alternifolia. The Melaleuca alternifolia is found in Australia (Southwest Queensland and New South Wales.) Tea Tree Oil should NEVER be taken (digested) internally – it's toxic. However, Tea Tree Oil is used topically for a variety of skin issues and other maladies.

What are the healing ingredients of tea tree oil?
Tea Tree Oil is composed of 98 compounds and 06 oil compositions. Tea Tree Oil has antifungal properties, antimicrobial properties, antiseptic properties, and inflammatory properties.

How does Tea Tree Oil work?
As I just stated, Tea Tree Oil has antifungal properties, antimicrobial properties, antiseptic properties, and inflammatory properties and they go after the bad guys to fight disease, infections, pain,…

What are some healing ways of Tea Tree Oil?

Here's a list of maladies treated by Tea Tree Oil:

- Acne
- Asthma (add a few drops to humidifier)
- Athlete's Foot
- Bad Breath (add a couple drops to water, swish and spit out)
- Colds (inhaling oils)
- Coughs (inhaling oils)
- Dandruff
- Herpes
- Insect Bites
- Itchiness
- Lice (add a few drops to shampoo)
- Mouthwash (add a couple drops to water, swish and spit out)
- Minor Cuts
- Psoriasis
- Rash
- Remove Ticks
- Ringworm
- Skin Tags
- Staph Infection
- Sunburn
- Toenail Fungus
- Warts

Where can I get some authentic Tea Tree Oil?
I've always found Tea Tree Oil at Walmart and no doubt it can be found at Walgreens, CVS, other drug stores, and other local stores.

WARNING: According to the American Cancer Society, ingesting tea tree oil has been reported to cause:
- Blood Cell Abnormalities
- Coma
- Confusion
- Diarrhea
- Drowsiness
- Hallucinations
- Severe Rash
- Unsteadiness
- Upset Stomach
- Vomiting
- Weakness

Tea Tree Oil should be **kept away from pets and children**. Tea tree oil should not be used in or around the mouth (DO NOT DIGEST).

For a safer product, SEE *Oil Of Oregano* in this Survival Book.

"Unbelievable Healing Ways Of Turpentine Oil!"

I thought I'd give you some great healthy data from the horse's mouth. I listened to all 03 audios and I gotta tell you. If you're concerned for your health right now and healthy future – **LISTEN to all these FREE audios**. Go to your computer and type-in the below information into the search bar.

Dr. Jennifer Daniels – *Turpentine: The Miracle Medicine And Candida Cleaner*

There are a few websites that come up. The website you're looking for is *One Radio Network (November 14, 2013)*. Scroll down and you'll find Dr. Jennifer Daniels audio interviews (as of 08 February 2015).

http://oneradionetwork.com/health/dr-jennnifer-daniels-turpentine-the-miracle-medicine-and-candida-cleaner-november-14-2013/

Before I let you go, I want to give you some turpentine remedies from the Old West. These turpentine remedies are from my Survival Book – ***239+ Texas Ranger, Pioneer, Old West,… Survival Tricks And More!* at https://www.survivalexpertblog.com/52-survival-books/** OK, let's start with *Horse Snake Bite Remedy*.

Horse Snake Bite Remedy: Trekking across the great wilderness, horses were bitten by rattlesnakes. And the Mormons had their own snake bite remedy. In his diary, William Clayton states: *"A number of horses have been bitten by rattlesnakes and one is dead. About nine o'clock Kendall one of my teamsters, brought one of the horses he drives into camp which had been bitten by a rattlesnake. His nose had begun to swell badly. We got some spirits of turpentine and bathed the wound, washed his face in salt and water and give him some snakes master root boiled in milk. He yet seems very sick."*

The horse died the next day. But Clayton himself states the remedy of snakes master root may have killed the horse due to an overdose of this plant. Clayton stated: *"Evening, Kennedy came to look at our horse and says that have given sufficient of the master root to kill four well horses."* Snake master root, also called milkwort is a plant used as a snake bite remedy via its rhizomes and roots. It's found in eastern North America.

Human Snake Bite Remedy: Those trekking Mormons always had the worry of venomous snakes along their trek westward. On 23 May 1847, 24-year old Nathaniel Fairbanks was tagged in the calf by a rattlesnake. His tongue began to feel prickly and numb, followed by stomach pains, dizziness,...

Coming to his aid, his Mormon comrades applied a mixture of tobacco juice & turpentine to the bite. Fairbanks also drank a mixture of alcohol & water. In a few hours he began feeling better.

Bruises And Aching Joints Remedy: To remedy bruises and joint aches, pioneers applied turpentine to the problem site.

Cold Remedy: Pioneers had their own cold and fever remedy. They used an ointment concoction of goose grease and turpentine. The exact application is unknown. Have you ever seen a goose with a cold? There you go!

"Healing Wonders Of Krill Oil!"

What is Krill Oil?

Krill oil is an extract from a species called Antarctic krill (*Euphausia superba*). The Antarctic krill is a small crustacean (small shrimp) that live in large schools, called swarms with numbers reaching 10,000-30,000 krills per cubic meter.

The krill feed on phytoplankton. The krill grows to 2.4 inches in length and weighs 0.071 ounces and it can live up to 06 years. The krill provides a bounty of both omega-3 fats eicosapentanoic acid (EPA) and docosahexanoic acid (DHA) oils.

What's the difference between Krill Oil and fish oil?

The krill provides a bounty of both omega-3 fats eicosapentanoic acid (EPA) and docosahexanoic acid (DHA) oils.

The EPA and DHA structure in krill oil makes the krill oil more absorbable than fish oil. Krill oil enters the body at the cellular level much better than fish oil easier.

Does Krill Oil contain any vitamins?

Krill oil contains vitamin E, vitamin A, and vitamin D.

a) Vitamin A is noted as an antioxidant which protects cells against cancer. This Vitamin slows the aging process as well as helping prevent night blindness, other eye problems, and skin disorders like acne. Vitamin A protects against colds, flu and infections.

b) Vitamin D is needed for calcium and phosphorous absorption and utilization. Necessary for growth, Vitamin D is especially important for normal growth and development of bones and teeth in children. Vitamin D is important in the prevention and treatment of osteoporosis, rickets, and hypocalcemia as well as enhancing immunity!

c) Vitamin E improves circulation, repairs tissue, and is useful in treating fibrocystic breast and premenstrual syndrome. Vitamin E promotes normal clotting and healing, reduces scarring from wounds, reduces blood pressure, aids in preventing cataracts, improves athletic performance, and aids in leg cramps!

Vitamin E prevents cell damage and the formation of free radicals as well as retards aging and may prevent age spots. Zinc is essential to maintain proper levels of Vitamin E in the blood.

What other healthy ingredients does Krill Oil contain?
Krill oil also provides canthaxanthin, a potent anti-oxidant. The anti-oxidant potency of krill oil compared to fish oil in terms of ORAC (Oxygen Radical Absorptance Capacity) values it was found to be 48 times more potent than fish oil.

Can Krill Oil help with bad cholesterol levels?
Studies have reported that krill oil is extremely effective in reducing LDL-cholesterol and the good HDL-cholesterol levels.

Can Krill Oil help to improve blood sugar levels?
Studies have reported that krill oil lowers blood sugar.

Can Krill Oil help with aches and pains?
Krill oil has been reported to remedy pain, aches and inflammation from rheumatoid arthritis.

Can Krill Oil help with other maladies?
In another study, Krill oil was reported to reduce PMS and dysmenorrhea. And it has been shown to be effective in the treatment of adult ADHD (Attention-Deficit Hyperactivity Disorder).

What are some other reported testimonials of Krill Oil?

- Alzheimer's Disease
- Antioxidant
- Arthritis
- Attention-Deficit Hyperactivity Disorder
- Cardiovascular
- Depression
- Diabetes
- Eye Health
- Mental Faculties (acuity, alertness, focus, memory)
- PMS
- Rheumatoid Arthritis
- Skin Health
- Weight-Loss

"The Super Healing Effects Of Oil Pulling!"

What the heck is Oil Pulling?
Oil Pulling is an ancient Ayurvedic dental application that has the user swishing a tablespoon of oil (coconut oil) in the mouth for approximately 15 - 20-minutes. Oil Pulling improves oral health and health throughout the body.

What are the many health benefits of Oil Pulling:
In the year 2000, the Surgeon General of the United States issued a report - *"Oral Health in America,"* noting the unknown unhealthy link between oral health and overall health.

The *"Oral Health in America"* Report is the *"silent factor promoting the onset of life-threatening diseases which are responsible for the deaths of millions of Americans each year."*

Your mouth is home to <u>BILLIONS</u> of bacteria, viruses, fungi, parasites,... and myriad other toxins. And strains of germs such as candida and streptococcus and their toxic waste products not only cause gum disease and tooth decay, but also contribute to serious and even debilitating health problems.

With the billions of bacteria, viruses, fungi, parasites,… and myriad other toxins in your mouth, your immune system is overburdened by factors such as excessive stress, poor diet, and environmental toxins, destructive organisms from your mouth can spread throughout the body. Once unleashed in the body, these toxins can generate secondary infections, chronic inflammation, and other persistent health problems.

The Mayo Clinic (Jacksonville, Florida -USA) staff lists the following diseases and conditions that may be caused or affected by oral health:
- Cardiovascular disease
- Endocarditis (infection of the inner lining of the heart)
- Premature birth and low birth weight
- Diabetes
- HIV/AIDS
- Eating disorders
- Osteoporosis
- Alzheimer's disease
- Immune system disorders

Last year I started reading at what is called Oil Pulling. Oil Pulling is simply swishing a few teaspoons of oil (coconut oil) in your mouth for 20-minutes each day. The 20-minutes of swishing the oil around in your mouth has a list of benefits. Back in April 2014, I tried Oil Pulling just 03-times, only 03-times for only 20-mintes each time and I got immediate relief from nasal congestion and bleeding gums.

That was my brief R & D. Now here's a list of the benefits of Oil Pulling:

- Arthritis
- Asthma
- Bad Breath
- Bleeding Gums
- Body Detox
- Boosts Immune System
- Clearer Mind
- Congestion
- Decreased Joint Pain
- Elimination Of Allergies
- Enhances Kidney Function
- Enhances Liver Function
- Gum Disease
- Gums Restored To Pink Color
- Hangover
- Headaches
- Improves Acne
- Improved Cardiovascular
- Improved Sleep
- Improves Skin Condition
- Increased Energy
- Increased Metabolism
- Jaw Soreness
- Migraines
- Nasal / Sinus Congestion
- TMJ

- Tooth Decay
- Vision Improvement
- Whiter Teeth

MOST IMPORTANT NOTE: After putting this segment together, I am convinced of the benefits of Oil Pulling and will start a schedule immediately.

Exactly how do I do Oil Pulling?
Oil Pulling is done by swishing a tablespoon full or two of oil in your mouth for 20 to 30 minutes after you get up in the morning. Oil Pulling is used with sunflower oil, olive oil, or coconut oil. Most prefer coconut oil. Why? Cause coconut oil has Anti-Bacteria, Anti-Fungal and Anti-Viral properties which gives your own immune system a better chance to improve your health cause now it can fight other bad guys throughout your body.

Are there any bad side-effects of Oil Pulling?
According to my research and experience, I myself have had no ill side-effects whatsoever with oil pulling using coconut oil. My best advice is to do your own research and seek advice from your personal health care physician.

YOU MUSE SEE *'Swishing Away Toothache Pain In Minutes'* at the end of the segment *'STOP Toothache Pain With This Super Oil.'*

"Weight-Loss Oils To The Rescue!"

Here's a list of oils that enhance weight-loss and why they work to help you lose that unwanted unhealthy extra weight. Let's start with *Avocado Oil*, but first let me tell you about some 'fats' you gotta know about so you understand why you can lose that unhealthy weight. Let me start with *Monounsaturated Fats*.

Essential Fatty Acids---They are substances that the body cannot manufacture and therefore must be supplied in the diet.

Fat---A body is composed of body fat and fat-free mass. Fat-free mass includes bone, body fluids, muscles and organs. Body fat is classified as essential fat or storage fat. Essential fat is needed for body function. This essential fat is stored in major body organs and tissues like bones, heart, intestines, kidneys, liver, lungs, muscles, spleen and throughout the central nervous system. Females have additional fat in the breast and pelvic region for child-bearing and other hormone-related functions.

a) **The Bad Fat:** The bad fat is excessive storage fat brought on by an unhealthy diet. Storage fat is the extra fat that accumulates in adipose cells (fat cells) around internal organs and beneath the skin surface.

91

Fat cells are with you forever. They expand (02 to 03 times) and contract as energy is stored and burned. Each fat gram consumed has twice the calories of a carbohydrate.

b) **Fat Calories:** Fat calories are harder to burn off than the same amount of calories from carbohydrates. Dietary fat is easily converted to body fat. On the other hand, only a small amount complex carbohydrates are converted to body fat. Saturated fats are high in cholesterol and increase blood cholesterol. Fat has 9 calories per gram compared to protein with 4 calories per gram and starches with 4 calories per gram. Want to lose weight? Reduce the fat in your diet.

Gram---A gram is a unit of weight. Many Nutritional Fact labels address   fat, cholesterol, sodium, carbohydrates, protein and sugar, in grams. Thirty grams is equal to one ounce or two tablespoons, or 1/8th cup.

So when you see a Nutritional Fact label that states 03 grams of saturated fat and there are 10 servings and you ate all 10 servings you just ate 30 grams of fat, or two tablespoons of fat, or 1/8th cup of fat. Doesn't seem like much but it surely is a great deal of fat, especially if you eat like this from day to day.

"HOW MUCH FAT IS IN YOUR FOOD? DO THE MATH!"

Use this formula to determine HOW MUCH FAT a product contains, before you buy it.

Step 1 -- Multiply 09 (number of calories per gram of fat) by the number of fat grams per serving stated on the label.

Step 2 -- Divide this number of total fat calories by the number of total calories per serving.

Step 3 -- Multiply your answer by 100.

Example: 09 times 04 (calories per gram of fat) = 36.
36 divided by 200 (total calories per serving) = .18
.18 times 100 = 18.
This package is 18% calories from fat (noodle soup).

The Bad -- Cholesterol:---Cholesterol's job is to carry fat through your blood vessels. Fat cannot travel through your blood vessels on its own because fat doesn't mix with water and water is a major ingredient in blood. Cholesterol does this very well and in a healthy way until there is too much fat content in your diet along with Bad Cholesterol. Read more about Cholesterol in Section 08.

The Ugly -- Blood Pressure (High):---Nearly 60 million Americans have high blood pressure or hypertension. When cholesterol build-up causes arteries to narrow, your heart pumps harder to push the blood through your arteries. Pressure on your arteries walls is stronger and High Blood Pressure\Hypertension is the result. Hypertension is a life-threatening disease.

Keys to CUTTING FAT & CALORIES IN COOKING:
- Trim fat before cooking.
- Roast or broil meat on a rack.
- Brown meat, then drain fat before continuing to cook in pan.
- Remove fat (skim from top) from stews or soups after chilling.
- Use low fat cooking methods such as bake, broil, microwave, roast, stir-fry, or braise.

Lipid---A lipid is a liquid fat or fatty substance.

Lipid Peroxidation---Lipid Peroxidation is the rancifying or spoiling of fatty substances.

Lipoprotein---Lipoprotein are packages of cholesterol, protein and triglycerides which circulate through the bloodstream.

Liver---The liver is the largest organ in the body. The liver secretes bile and acts in the formation of blood and in the metabolism of carbohydrates, fats, proteins, minerals and vitamins. The liver also removes worn-out cells from the blood and reprocesses their red pigment hemoglobin.

Mediterranean Diet---The Mediterranean Diet is a diet low in meat, but high in cereal, fruit, grain, legumes, monounsaturated fats, nuts, and vegetables. Recent French Study found that the Mediterranean Diet after a heart attack was 70 percent more life-saving than the Standard American Diet (low-fat diet-less than 30 percent fat calories). Some Harvard Researchers favor the Mediterranean Diet over the Standard American Diet.

A research effort, called the Seven Countries Study, examined 12,763 men ages 40 through 59 in the Netherlands, Finland, Italy, Greece, Croatia and Serbia, Japan, and the United States.

Ten years after their initial screening, the study reported several important results:
- Mediterranean groups had lower death rates from all causes than the northern European and American groups.
- Lower mortality from coronary heart disease in the Mediterranean countries.

- Men at the peak of their lives (45 years) have longer life expectancies in Greece than in any other European or North American country despite their high tobacco consumption, low exercise level, and modest health-care system.

The Mediterranean Diet is based on traditional eating patterns evolving over centuries in Greece, Italy, North Africa, Southern France, Spain and several Middle Eastern nations. All share a general pattern of cooking and ingredients. The diet is rich in fruits, vegetables, legumes and grains.

The principal fat is olive oil! Lean red meat is eaten only a few times a month and in small portions. Eating foods from animal sources - namely dairy products, fish, and poultry is low to moderate. Wine is drunk with meals. Plenty of crusty country-style bread is enjoyed with each meal.

The major fat used in the Mediterranean Diet is olive oil! Olive oil is primarily a monounsaturated fat, which is noted to lower harmful low-density lipoprotein (LDL) blood cholesterol and may increase good high-density lipoprotein (HDL) blood cholesterol. Olive oil isn't the only key to a healthy diet.

Here are some Mediterranean Eating Tips:

- Switch to olive oil (extra virgin).
- Avoid butter and margarine. There is nothing wrong with putting olive oil on toast or whole grain bread.
- Cut meat consumption. If you do eat meat, ensure it's lean. Try small portions of poultry or fish with plenty of vegetables.
- INCREASE fruit and vegetable consumption.
- Eat plenty of whole grain bread. The darker the better (ingredients not burnt).
- Eat a salad at the beginning and end of each meal.
- Wine at each dinner meal. It's been noted that a couple glasses of wine each day may protect against coronary heart disease.

People in the Mediterranean have been noted to develop far less heart disease than Americans, even though they drink, smoke, and even consume as much or more saturated fat than Americans! What are they doing different? Their diet consists of an oil they use on their vegetables, grain-rich dishes, and meats. They even dip their bread in it! It's olive oil! Yes, olive oil.

Medium Chain Triglycerides (MCT)---MCT's have been used in medicine for almost 40 years for patients who have difficulty digesting or absorbing nutrients or who need a rapidly available source of energy.

MCT's are 1/3 to 1/2 the size of long chain triglycerides (LCT's) which are found in virtually all oils in the foods we eat like butter, margarine, animal fats and vegetable oils. MCT's are much more water-soluble than LCT's meaning there are rapidly burned for energy!

LCT's (fat) on the other hand, may be stored in the body and utilized at a later time. MCT's may be a great diet replacement for LCT's.

Monounsaturated Fats---Monounsaturated fats (good fat) help lower bad LDL cholesterol, blood pressure and protect the arteries from arteriosclerosis (clogging of the arteries). Monounsaturated fats are found in foods like avocadoes, canola oil, olives, olive oil, peanuts and peanut oil.

OBESITY: Obesity is the state of having an excessive amount of fat on the body. Twenty percent over your maximum healthy weight according to your height and build is considered obese.

Approximately 58 million adults are considered overweight or obese. Extra pounds raise your risk of developing diabetes, heart disease, stroke and some forms of cancer. In 1995 300,000 deaths resulted from overweight-related diseases.

According to Jane Schultz of the Snack Foods Association in Alexandria, Virginia the average American ate a whopping 22 pounds of salty snacks in 1994 compared to 17.5 pounds in 1988.

No wonder the majority of Americans are obese. First, we'll take a look at what the Chinese are doing to stay slim!

Chinese consume 300 more calories per day than Americans, yet they have lower rates of obesity, heart disease, and cancer. What's their secret? The Chinese diet consist of high fiber, non-fat, antioxidant-rich fruits and vegetables which is only 15% of calories from fat.

This diet reflects their low rates of cancer, heart disease and obesity. The Chinese also exercise a great deal more than Americans. While Americans are driving or riding everywhere they go, even very short distances, Chinese are bicycling everywhere they go!

WARNING: Don't be fooled by the Chinese restaurants in the United States. Many do not serve the healthy, authentic Chinese foods found in China. Ask for nutritional facts of each meal before you order!

Polyunsaturated Fat---Polyunsaturated fats may lower the cholesterol in the blood. Sources of polyunsaturated fats are corn, safflower, soybean and sunflower seed oils.

Saturated Fat---Saturated fats are fats that harden at room temperature and may raise blood cholesterol levels. Saturated fats are found in most animal and some vegetable products like butter, coconut oil, cream, palm oil and whole milk products.

Trans Fatty Acids---Trans fatty acids are created when liquid vegetable oils are hydrogenated, a process where bubbling hydrogen through the oil. This is done to make the oils more solid and increase their shelf life. It is noted that processed foods containing *"hydrogenated oils"* should be avoided.

Triglycerides---They are the most common fat molecule found in fatty tissue. The body turns dietary fats into triglycerides, which are a storage form of fat. Triglycerides can be broken down for energy in times of need. Triglycerides in excess team up with cholesterol and other substances to clog the arteries and cause heart attacks and strokes.

"LOSE FAT BY EATING FATS!"

Avocado Oil---Avocado Oil is produced from fresh pressed avocadoes. Avocado oil is noted to be bountiful in rich in monounsaturated fats. Healthy monounsaturated fats are noted to help improve cholesterol levels and hold off that hunger when you're really not hungry.

Avocado oil also provides needed vitamin B and vitamin E. Add avocado oil to those healthy salads, breads, and glycemic approved pasta recipes.

a) All the B Vitamins aid to maintain healthy eyes, hair, liver, mouth, and muscle tone in the gastrointestinal tract, nerves, and skin. B-Complex Vitamins are coenzymes involved in energy production. B-Complex Vitamins may be useful to combat depression or anxiety. The B Vitamins should be taken together. Follow the recommended dosage and instructions from the label and as per your doctor's instructions.

b) Vitamin E improves circulation, repairs tissue, and is useful in treating fibrocystic breast and premenstrual syndrome. Vitamin E promotes normal clotting and healing, reduces scarring from wounds, reduces blood pressure, aids in preventing cataracts, improves athletic performance, and aids in leg cramps!

Vitamin E prevents cell damage and the formation of free radicals as well as retards aging and may prevent age spots. Zinc is essential to maintain proper levels of Vitamin E in the blood.

Canola Oil---Canola Oil comes the extraction of a variety of several rape plants from the broccoli family. Canola Oil provides omega-6 and omega-3 fats with a good ratio of 02.5 to 01 ratio. According to a study in Experimental Biology and Medicine, people who achieve a dietary ratio similar to this have been able to battle arthritis, asthma, and cancer more effectively.

Canola Oil is also noted to be rich in alpha-linolenic acid (ALA) which is an essential omega-3 fatty acid that may play a role in **weight maintenance**. Canola has a high smoke point and can be used for frying, and other cooking recipes because of its neutral taste.

Coconut Oil---Coconut oil got a bad rap years ago. Sixty-five percent of coconut oil's saturated fat is mostly made up of medium-chain triglycerides (MCTs). Populations like Polynesian Puka Puka and Tokelau islanders that consume most of their fat from coconut oil have low rates of heart disease!

Coconut oil, unlike other oils, is **less likely to attribute to obesity**. Why? Your body easily converts coconut oil into energy rather than depositing calories as body fat.

Coconut oil also kills germs! It contains anti-microbial components like mother's milk. The Polynesian Puku Puku and Tokelau islanders live in an environment ideal for parasites. They're protected from parasites by the coconut oil in their diet.

It may be wise to avoid processed products like margarine, chips, and cookies that have trans-fatty acids. According to a study by Dr. Walter Willett, of Harvard University, trans-fatty acids double the risk of heart attack. Trans-fatty acids may also contribute to cancer, diabetes, and obesity.

Read the contents before you purchase the product. Look for *"partially hydrogenated oils."* If you read this, AVOID IT!

MOST IMPORTANT NOTE: Recent reports indicate that a simple thing like consuming Coconut Oil may STOP and REVERSE Alzheimer's disease. I encourage you to view videos on YouTube and do your own research.

Flaxseed & Flaxseed Oil: In 1909, the average U.S. person consumed approximately 125 grams of fat per day.

Today the average person in the U.S. consumes approximately 175 grams of fat, an increase of 40 percent or about 50 extra pounds per year and increasing! Of the total increase in the consumption of fats and oils, shortening, margarine, refined salad oil and cooking oils account for fifty percent.

This increase in fat over the years is undoubtedly linked to the increase in degenerative diseases. In order to extend the shelf life of many products, essential fatty acids (good fat) have been purposely processed out of most foods.

This is profitable for the manufacturer, but UNHEALTHY to the American consumer - YOU! Approximately 80% of Americans are deficient in essential fatty acids. Flax seed has a high content of essential fatty acids. Flax seed supplies the body with needed essential fatty acids, is richer in Omega-3's than fish oil, and packs more fiber ounce for ounce than oat bran!

Listed below are some observed benefits of flax seed:
- Seriously ill cancer patients were treated with flax seed oil and low-fat cottage cheese by Dr. Johanna Budwig. Over a period of approximately 90 days, tumors gradually receded. Symptoms of anemia, cancer, diabetes, and liver dysfunction were completely alleviated!

- According to a study in Great Britain by Dr. Sinclair, a relative deficiency of the essential fatty acids plays an important part in the causes of arteriosclerosis, coronary thrombosis, diabetes mellitus, hypertension, multiple sclerosis, and certain forms of malignant diseases!

- Dr. J.R. Vane shared the 1982 Nobel Prize for Medicine for his work proving how the metabolism of Omega-3 fatty acids helped prevent heart problems.

- A U.S. physician, Dr. Donald Rudin, discovered that Omega-3 fatty acid deficiency is the basic cause of major mental illness because fatty acids provide the substance upon which niacin and other B Vitamins act to form the prostaglandin-3 series tissue hormones which are special mission fatty acids that regulate neurocircuits through the whole body.

The Food and Drug Administration (FDA) has recently entered into a 03-year, $2 million contract with the National Cancer Institute (NCI) to research the effect of flax seed on various health concerns.

The FDA will conduct experiments confirming flaxseed's role in fat and cholesterol metabolism, bone mineralization, and the immune system. This research will make flaxseed one of the most intensively-studied nutrients used in any food product.

Flax seeds are a great source of healthy soluble and insoluble fiber as well as protein. Just 1/4 cup (50 grams) of flax seed provides 20 grams of fiber. Remember fiber is noted to ameliorate, heal, or prevent:

- Colon cancer
- Constipation
- Diverticulosis
- Hemorrhoids
- Improves blood sugar metabolism
- Lowers blood pressure
- Lowers cholesterol
- Protects against other cancers
- Rectal cancer
- **Weight loss**
- Much more

Olive Oil---Olive oil varies in quality. The term *"virgin"* is loosely applied. Originally it meant that the oil was from the first pressing of the fruit, as opposed to the second or third pressing. Olive oil when unrefined has a greenish tinge and a pungent flavor. It is preferred to refined oils because the health qualities are intact.

I've found that Extra Virgin Italian Olive Oil (cold pressed), is one of the best bets for a quality oil.

Many studies have shown that populations using large amounts of olive oil like Italy and Greece have lower heart disease and stroke. Olive oil is rich in Vitamin E and a known antioxidant. Olive oil is linked to longevity - olive trees have been known to live as long as 3,000 years!

Olive oil may be one of the best choices when cooking with oils. Olive oil IS NOT saturated fat but is a monounsaturated fatty acid, which is stable at high temperatures and less prone to oxidation than other vegetable oils. Extra Virgin Oil is probably your best choice of all the other oils.

All cooking oils are 100% fat. Vegetable oils contain a combination of saturated, monounsaturated, and polyunsaturated fats in varying proportions. There is no such thing as a saturated-fat-free oil or one containing purely monounsaturated or polyunsaturated fat.

One study may contradict another study concerning the health benefits or negative results of one oil or another. One fact is agreed upon by most studies. Consuming products that have saturated fat has been linked to a very long list of diseases.

The bottom line is to cut the fat. If oils are required for cooking, cook with monounsaturated fats since studies are still finding their beneficial affects towards health for you above polyunsaturated fats.

According to the American Journal of Nutrition, smelling olive oil may help you **lose weight**. Why? Cause it increases the feelings of being full.

During a 02-day study, 11 male subjects were fed low-fat yogurt, and half of those subjects were fed yogurt mixed with fat-free olive oil extract. After the snack, German researchers measured the men's brain activity.

It turns out the group that ate yogurt with the olive oil extract had increased blood flow in brain, particularly the areas of the brain associated with fat consumption. Why? It's due to the scent of olive oil, which help you feel full.

Macadamia Nut Oil---Approximately 80% of the fat in macadamia nuts is monounsaturated fats meaning it will help you **lose unhealthy extra weight**. Macadamia nut oil also has a good percentage of omega-3s fatty acids. It is also a great source of phytosterols which is a plant-derived compound that has been associated with decreased cancer risk.

Macadamia oil has a medium to high smoke point so you can use it for stir frying healthy and tasty vegetables, and you can bake with it. Also use the buttery tasty macadamia oil and use it on and salads.

Peanut Oil---Peanut oil has a good bounty of monounsaturated which as you already know can help **reduce your appetite while promoting weight loss.** A study out of the University of California, Irvine, found that this particular type of fat may help to your boosts memory.

Peanut oil is very tasty and has a high smoke point. Peanut oil is famous for frying whole thawed turkeys and can be used for frying and baking.

Walnut Oil---Walnut Oil has a rich roasted nutty taste. Walnut oil is rich in polyunsaturated fatty acids. Walnuts have more omega-3 fatty acids than any other nut.

Those polyunsaturated fatty acids may **increase diet-induced calorie burn and resting metabolic rate.** Walnut Oil has a low smoke point which isn't considered the best oil for cooking. However, Walnut Oil can be used in salad dressings.

"ARE YOU OBESE? - BODY MASS INDEX (BMI) FORMULA"

How to calculate your own BMI.

STEP ONE: Multiply your weight in pounds by 0.45 to get kilograms.
Example: 140 pounds X .45 = 63 kilograms.

STEP TWO: Multiply your height in inches by 0.025 to get meters.
Example: 67 inches X 0.025 = 1.675 meters

STEP THREE: Square the answer in STEP TWO to get your height measurement in meters.
Example: 1.675 X 1.675 = 2.805

STEP FOUR: Divide your weight in kg (STEP ONE) by your height in meters (STEP THREE).
Example: 63 divided by 2.805 = 22.45.

RESULTS AND RECOMMENDATIONS:

A BMI of 19 to 25 is healthy.
A BMI of 27 to 30 means you are at risk and it is advisable to lose weight (see your doctor).
NOTE: BMI is a standard measure of body fat used to monitor obesity.

"WHAT IS YOUR HEALTHY WEIGHT?"

Height	Weight Upper Limits	Target Weight
4' 10"	119 pounds	109 pounds
4' 11"	124 pounds	114 pounds
5 feet	128 pounds	118 pounds
5' 01"	132 pounds	121 pounds
5' 02"	136 pounds	125 pounds
5' 03"	141 pounds	130 pounds
5' 04"	145 pounds	133 pounds
5' 05"	150 pounds	138 pounds
5' 06"	155 pounds	143 pounds
5' 07"	159 pounds	146 pounds
5' 08"	164 pounds	151 pounds
5' 09"	169 pounds	154 pounds
5' 10"	174 pounds	160 pounds
5' 11"	179 pounds	165 pounds
6 feet	184 pounds	169 pounds
6' 01"	189 pounds	174 pounds
6' 02"	194 pounds	178 pounds
6' 03"	200 pounds	184 pounds
6' 04"	205 pounds	189 pounds

Source: American Health Foundation.

Weight Loss – Refers to weight loss during a period of time where a routine of exercise, diet and other factors are incorporated. See your doctor prior to initiating any weight-loss program. See my Survival Book ***169+ Lose It Or Else Accelerated Weight-Loss Facts, Tricks, And More!*** at http://www.loseitorelseweightloss.com/

"The Mediterranean Diet!"

The Mediterranean Diet is a diet low in meat, but high in cereal, fruit, grain, legumes, monounsaturated fats, nuts, and vegetables. Recent French Study found that the Mediterranean Diet after a heart attack was 70 percent more life-saving than the Standard American Diet (low-fat diet-less than 30 percent fat calories). Some Harvard Researchers favor the Mediterranean Diet over the Standard American Diet.

A research effort, called the Seven Countries Study, examined 12,763 men ages 40 through 59 in the Netherlands, Finland, Italy, Greece, Croatia and Serbia, Japan, and the United States.

Ten years after their initial screening, the study reported several important results:

- Mediterranean groups had lower death rates from all causes than the northern European and American groups.
- Lower mortality from coronary heart disease in the Mediterranean countries.
- Men at the peak of their lives (45 years) have longer life expectancies in Greece than in any other European or North American country despite their high tobacco consumption, low exercise level, and modest health-care system.

The Mediterranean Diet is based on traditional eating patterns evolving over centuries in Greece, Italy, North Africa, Southern France, Spain and several Middle Eastern nations. All share a general pattern of cooking and ingredients. The diet is rich in fruits, vegetables, legumes, and grains. The principal fat is olive oil! Lean red meat is eaten only a few times a month and in small portions. Eating foods from animal sources - namely dairy products, fish, and poultry is low to moderate.

Wine is drunk with meals. Plenty of crusty country-style bread is enjoyed with each meal. The major fat used in the Mediterranean Diet is olive oil! Olive oil is primarily a monounsaturated fat, which is noted to lower harmful low-density lipoprotein (LDL) blood cholesterol and may increase good high-density lipoprotein (HDL) blood cholesterol. Olive oil isn't the only key to a healthy diet.

Mediterranean Diet Eating Tips:
- Switch to olive oil (extra virgin).

- Avoid butter and margarine. There is nothing wrong with putting olive oil on toast or whole grain bread.

- Cut meat consumption. If you do eat meat, ensure it's lean. Try small portions of poultry or fish with plenty of vegetables.

- INCREASE fruit and vegetable consumption.

- Eat plenty of whole grain bread. The darker the better (ingredients not burnt).

- Eat a salad at the beginning and end of each meal.

- Wine at each dinner meal. It's been noted that a couple glasses of wine each day may protect against coronary heart disease.

"UNADVERTISED BONUS HEALING!"

The Amazing Wonders Of Cold Water Cures!

Cold Water Cures: If there is one thing I hate more than 08-legged spiders, it's cold frigid water. I can still hold my own when it comes to cold weather to include being soaking wet with cold water (surface or submerged) but I just have a lot of *"Art Of Suffering"* bad miserable memories (military) when it comes to cold water, cold days, cold swamps, staying soaking wet for days,... Anyway, did you know plain ol' cold water has some **very beneficial healthy effects**?

According to Gurudev Khar Khalsa, a noted Sat Nam Rasayan Healer and Kundalini Yoga Teacher from Los Angeles, California: *"Cold Water Massage Therapy is one of the healthiest and most inexpensive of therapies. Simply massage the body with almond oil before taking a shower. Shower in cold water until your body temperature rises and no longer feels cold, but toasty and warm. Make sure the bathroom is heated. Never get out of a cold shower into a cold room."*

And here's list maladies remedied by cold water and complimentary benefits of taking cold showers - Brrrrrrrrrrrrrrrrrrrr:
- Acne
- Allergies

115

- Anxiety Attacks
- Asthma
- Awake
- Blood Cholesterol Lower
- Blood Circulation
- Blood Pressure Reduced
- Blood Sugar Lowered
- Body Feels Warmer
- Body Odor Eliminated
- Calming Effect
- Cleanses Circulatory System
- Clearer Mind
- Complexion
- Concentration Improvement
- Depression Eliminated
- Dry Skin
- Eliminates Poisons & Toxins
- Energy
- Feelings Of Euphoria
- Five Senses Improved
- Flushes Organs
- Focus Improvement
- Hair Improvement
- Headaches Eliminated
- Heart Problems
- Heightened Awareness
- Immune System Booster
- Learning Improvement

- Less\No Colds
- Less\No Flu
- Leg Bloating\Pain,...
- Libido Improvement
- Mental Faculties Improved
- Migraines Eliminated
- Mood Improvement
- Muscle Cramps
- Pain
- Panic Attacks
- Positive Thoughts
- Pulse Rate Lower
- Rashes
- Refreshed
- Skin Improvement
- Sinusitis
- Sleep Improvement
- Strengthens Nervous System
- Strengthens Mucous Membranes
- Stress Buster
- Sweating Reduced
- Utility Bill Reduced
- Zest For Life

I've told you before that the **BLOOD RULES!** It's apparent to me that cold showers get the blood really moving thus the many benefits of plain ol' *Cold Water C*

"Want More Proof? Then Read This:"

Lake Baikal Fountain Of Youth: Lake Baikal is located in Siberia Russia, and it's the oldest and deepest freshwater lake (01-mile) in the world and complimented with 27 islands. It holds more water than all 05 Great Lakes in the Unites States combined. And many Russians swear it may be a fountain of youth. Let's start with *Curative Mineral Baths*.

a) Curative Mineral Baths: Whether you know it or not your own body is made up of many minerals which are needed for a healthy vibrant life. And minerals can be absorbed via baths - hot baths that open your skin's pours. Over 800 people a week go to Goryachinsks, a hot springs resort on Baikal's eastern shore. There, its patrons lazily soak in bathtubs filled with hot mineral waters straight from Baikal's underground hot springs. Many swear that Baikal's hot springs cured their sickly maladies.

b) Rejuvenating Waters: Lake Baikal's Siberian waters are killer cold. Its waters invite hypothermia with open arms. But on the other side of the coin, it's waters may be the Fountain Of Youth! Yuri and Sasha take part in the traditional Russian *banya*. Banya is bathing in a hot steam bath followed by a dip through a ice hole into super cold water. As Yuri brags *"Baikal makes you feel young again, like baby!"* Sasha adds *"Like you have milk in blood!"* (Taken from National Geographic - June 1992)

"Want Even More Proof? Then Read This:"

Back Pain Remedy: One of the crew members – Bratton (1805 – Lewis & Clark Expedition), was suffering from severe back pain. His back pain was so severe he had trouble just sitting up. So Captain Clark used an Indian application that actually healed Bratton's back problem. A 04-foot deep pit was dug out. A fire built inside the pit with rocks added to retain heat. Horsemint tea was added with Bratton sitting in the pit enveloped in the steam.

After several minutes in this sweat bath, Bratton was carried away and submerged in cold water. After a quick cold dip, he was returned to the home-made wet sauna bath. The repeated hot-cold, hot-cold treatment was repeated several times. After several applications, Bratton was wrapped in a blanket. His back pain improved the next day and he soon recovered completely.

1st Note: Horsemint includes several coarse aromatic plants like Mentha Longifolia.

2nd Note: This is a perfect example of an alternative medicine called Hydrotherapy. Here's a quote from the Gettysburg Program: ****"*Hydrotherapy is the use of water, ice, steam and hot and cold temperatures to maintain and **restore health.***

Treatments include full body immersion, steam baths, saunas, sitz baths, colonic irrigation and the application of hot and\or cold compresses. Hydrotherapy is effective for treating a wide range of conditions and can easily be used in the home as part of a self-care program."

"Want Some More Proof? Then Read This:"

Here's a true story how cold water can preserve the body and defy the sure-grip of death!

Cold Water Diving Reflex - They're Still Alive: Folks, one of the most unforgiving environments are frigid cold weather environments. Worse yet are killer cold water environments. The human body is not designed to hold-up in cold weather environments for any length of time or even short periods.

Once the core temperature drops below 98.6 degrees Fahrenheit - problems arise and get worse real quick the lower the body temperature drops. Simple shivering is a sign of hypothermia.

As I said, killer cold water environments are the worst. But there may be a way to bring back the dead, it's called *cold water diving reflex*. Let me go back in time and tell you a true story so you can better understand *cold water diving reflex*.

Several years ago, during the cold winter months in Fargo, North Dakota, an 11-year old boy with his sled was having fun like any other boy with his sled. The boy and his sled were over frozen water when he fell through the ice.

Fargo Rescue and other nearby departments were soon dispatched to the scene. Rescue workers deployed their boats into the water, breaking the ice and probing for the boy's body with grappling poles.

As more and more minutes went by, one would think that there was no hope for the young boy. But the rescue workers knew something most people are unaware of - it's called *cold water diving reflex*.

Cold water diving reflex not only retards the metabolism but puts the body's main organs in suspended animation to hold-off death! The multiple rescue workers were betting that if they found the boy real soon, *cold water diving reflex* would help them save the boy.

After 45 minutes under water, the boy was finally hooked - they found him. He was brought into the boat where they brought him to shore. His body temperature was only 77-degrees - he was dead dead!

Immediate CPR was applied to the boy on the way to the hospital. The paramedics revived the boy! At the hospital, the young boy made a full recovery! He was under the frigid water for 45-minutes and survived! He survived because of *cold water diving reflex*!

Now I'm not sure if *cold water diving reflex* applies only to children only or if it also apples to adults. This subject RFIR.

If you know any firemen, paramedics, doctors,... ask them and let me know what they say.

Now you understand why I keep telling you *"NEVER give-up, there's always a solution."* Before I end this subject, I want to give you some data on hypothermia survival and ice support thickness.

"Hypothermia Water Survival Table"

Water Temperature	Exhaustion & Max Time	Unconscious Survival Time
32.5 F	15-min	15-45 min
32.5-40 F	15-30min	30-90 min
40-50 F	30-60min	01-03 hrs
50-60 F	01-02hrs	01-06 hrs
60-70 F	02-07hrs	02-40 hrs
70-80 F	03-12hrs	03 hours+

NOTE: Other considerations are the survivor's swimming abilities, predators, prior cold injuries, other injuries, available flotation equipment or floating debris, weather conditions, survivor's attitude, and other survivors present and their status (above considerations).

"Ice Support Measurements!"

You & Equipment Weigh ??? -	Ice Should Be
One survivor - no equipment	02-inches thick
Group of Survivors in a file	03-inches thick
Car or snowmobile (02 tons)	7.5-inches thick
Light truck (02.5 tons)	08-inches thick
Medium truck (03.5 tons)	10-inches thick
Heavy truck (09 tons)	12-inches thick
10 tons of weight	15-inches thick
25 tons of weight	20-inches thick

NOTE: Before you venture on frozen ice (lakes, ponds...), insure you see the local Forest Ranger for best and up-to-date safe ice-thickness measurements.

If you're in a survival environment, <u>walk around</u> the frozen water obstacle.

"More Unadvertised BONUS Healing For YOU!"

THANK YOU FOR GETTING THIS SURVIVAL BOOK! SO HERE'S A **BONUS BONUS FOR YOU!** Here are 02 more Oils that are very worthy of your attention. They are direct quotes from my latest published Survival Book - *"99+ International Cancer Preventers, Cancer Fighters, Cancer Killers And More!"*

I'm going to tell you about the Healing Wonders of:
- **Frankincense Oil**
- **Myrrh Oil**

Let's start with *Frankincense Oil*.

Frankincense Oil: Frankincense is mentioned 68-times in the Bible and is also called *"The King Of Oils."* We all know the story from the Bible of the Three Wise Men. The Three Wise Men arrived in Bethlehem (southern region of Judea) shortly after the birth of Jesus.

The Three Wise Men presented Jesus with 03 gifts. Gold, Frankincense and Myrrh. Frankincense Oil comes from the *Boswellia sacra* tree and from similar species of trees (Ethiopia, Somalia, Oman and Yemen). The use of Frankincense is recorded as far back as 3,000 B.C.!

A single *Boswellia sacra* tree can produce a couple pounds of resin each year and the trees can live for hundreds of years.

126

Frankincense Oil is now more popular than ever as an alternative medicine to fight cancers and other minor and major maladies. Frankincense can be used for aroma therapy, consumed and applied to the skin to remedy a variety of maladies like:

- Acne
- Anti-aging
- Antiseptic
- Anxiety
- Arthritis
- Bad breath
- Bloating
- Boils
- Bowel movements
- Bronchitis
- Cancer fighter
- Cancer Killer (Apoptosis)
- Cancer (stops cancer from spreading)
- Cancer (stop cancer cell growth)
- Cavities
- Chronic colitis
- Crohn's Disease
- Cold
- Constipation
- Coughing
- Depression
- Digestive disorders
- Dispel negative feelings
- Dry skin

- Eczema
- Enhance mental faculties (see 2nd Note)
- Fatigue
- Fingernail rejuvenation
- Flu
- Flush out excess water
- Headaches
- Improve memory
- Increases blood flow
- Indigestion
- Infections
- Insect bites
- Irritable Bowel Syndrome
- Irritated skin
- Leaky gut syndrome
- Menopause symptoms
- Mouth sores
- Mouthwash
- Mood enhancer
- Mood swings
- Muscle aches
- Nausea
- Overall wellness
- Pain killer
- PMS
- Promotes relaxation
- Promotes sleep
- Razor bumps
- Reduce inflammation

- Reducing scars
- Regulate menstrual cycle
- Rejuvenate feet
- Rejuvenate hands
- Relieve anxiety
- Rheumatoid arthritis
- Scars
- Skin elasticity
- Skin imperfections
- Skin rejuvenation
- Skin tone
- Slow signs of aging
- Speed up healing
- Stomach aches
- Strengthen gums
- Strengthen hair roots
- Strengthens immune system
- Stretch marks
- Stop bleeding of minor wounds
- Toothaches (see *Clove Oil*)
- Tooth decay
- Uterine health
- Wrinkle fighter

1st Note: Frankincense Oil can be taken orally (adults only). A single drop of Frankincense Oil added to a carrier (tablespoon of coconut oil, or honey, or water…) should be considered safe.

2nd Note: Back in October & November 2016, I conducted my own R & D on Frankincense Oil. Every day, I applied a few drops to the back of my neck and massaged it in. I found that **MY MENTAL FACULTIES INCREASED LIKE NEVER BEFORE**.

Let me give you an example. People would ask me a question and in a split split second I was already spitting out the answer.

I answered their questions so fast like I already knew what they were going to ask me!! I got some weird looks too! I even surprised myself. Never have I ever answered questions so fast. **Don't believe me?** You try it under your Doctors OK. Since then, I have stopped using the Frankincense Oil.

About a week after I stopped applying Frankincense Oil to the back of my neck, my mental faculties returned to 'normal' – retarded state. I plan to continue my R & D after I re-publish this Survival Book (early May 2017).

WARNING: Frankincense Oil is not recommended for pregnant women or nursing mothers.

WAIT WAIT WAIT!!! I'm not done yet. Below are some FREE videos from YouTube you gotta check out.

Essential Oils As Medicine:
Essential Oils Guide (00:35:12)--------YouTube

Frankincense, Magical Healing Essential
Oils. [Young Living] (00:09:59)--------YouTube

Frankincense Stimulates Apoptosis
(Cancer Cell Death) Pt2w/Ant-Aging!
Essential Oil Video (00:20:04)---------YouTube

Frankincense Testimonial (00:02:11)----YouTube

Uses And Benefits Of
Frankincense (00:07:20)---------------YouTube

Myrrh Oil: Myrrh is mentioned 152-times in the Bible
and botanically known as *"Commiphora myrrha."* We all
know the story from the Bible of the Three Wise Men.

The Three Wise Men arrived in Bethlehem (southern
region of Judea) shortly after the birth of Jesus. The
Three Wise Men presented Jesus with 03 gifts.

Gold, Frankincense and Myrrh. Myrrh Oil is processed
from the resin of the Commiphora myrrha tree (Horn of
Africa & Middle East). Myrrh Oil has been used for at
least 5,000 years. Myrrh is related to Frankincense.

Myrrh Oil and Frankincense Oil may be the most popular
oils in the world.

Myrrh Oil can be used for aroma therapy, consumed and
applied to the skin to remedy a variety of maladies
like:
• Antidepressant

- Antimicrobial
- Anti-tumor
- Antiviral
- Anxiety
- Arthritis
- Athlete's Foot
- Blood circulation
- Colds
- Cough
- Cramps
- Diabetes
- Diarrhea
- Eczema
- Fever
- Food Poisoning
- Gas relief
- Gingivitis
- Healing wounds
- Immune booster
- Itching
- Laryngitis
- Measles
- Mood Swings
- Mouth ulcers
- Mumps
- Normalizes menstruation
- Phyorrhoea (inflammation of the gums)
- Premature aging
- Ringworm

- Scars
- Strenghthens gums
- Thrush

Follow the recommended dosage and instructions from the label and as per your doctor's instructions.

WARNING: Pregnant women should not consume Myrrh Oil. Consult your doctor.

More Survival Kindle E-Books And Survival Paperback Books For YOU!

Joseph A. Laydon Jr. (MSG Ret. Army) is the author and owner of Intensive Research Information Services And Products (IRISAP). Joseph has been writing "*self-reliance*" orientated data since 1991 and since July 2012 has been re-publishing his works via Kindle E-Books and Kindle Paperback Books. He has self-published more than **100+ Survival Books** (Kindle E-Books and Kinde Paperback Books). Below is a list of all his Survival Books and you can see these books by simply going to the website listed below for detailed descriptions and videos. See "*About The Author.*"

- **Kindle E-Books:**----------www.survivalexpertblog.com/52-survival-books/

- **Kindle Paperback:**-------www.survivalexpertblog.com/52-survival-books/

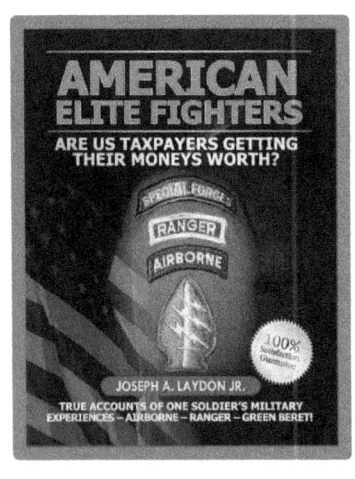 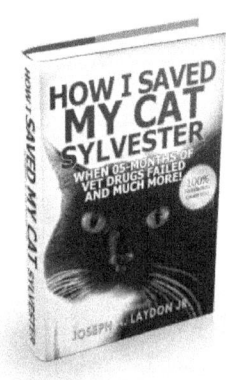 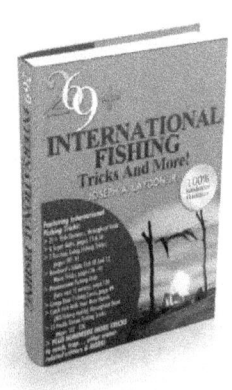

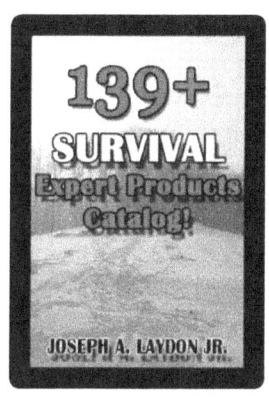

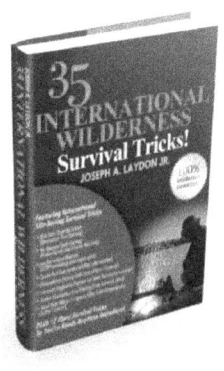

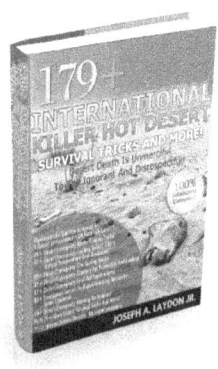

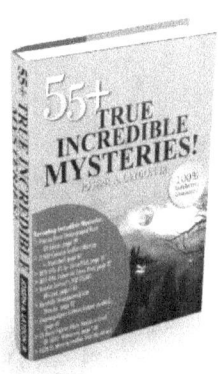

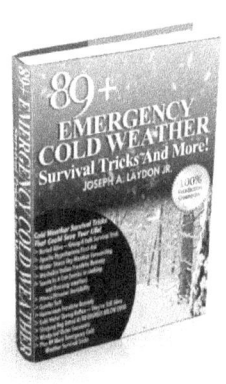

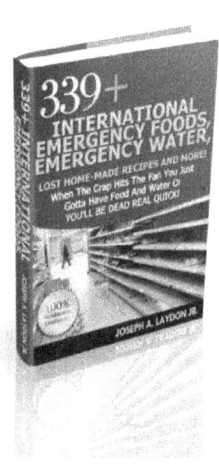

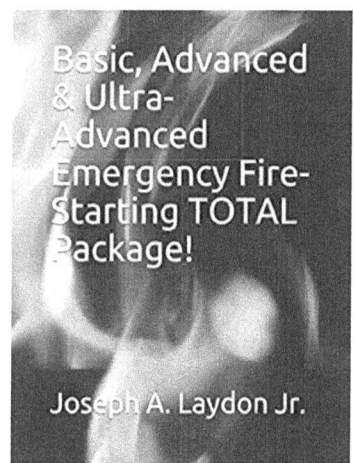

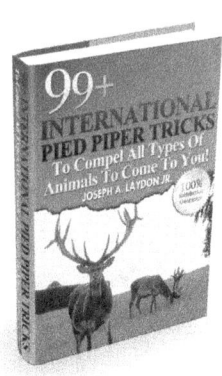

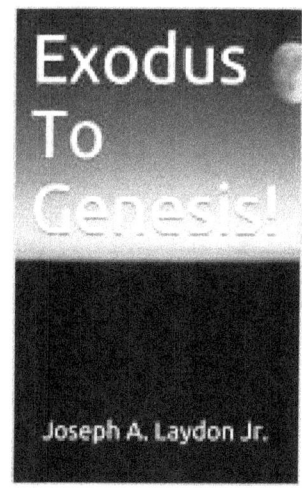

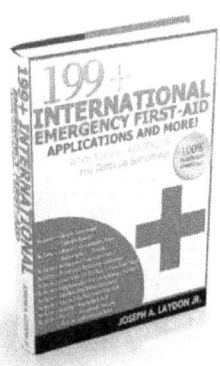

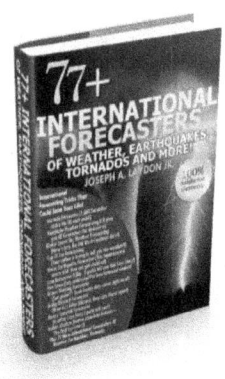

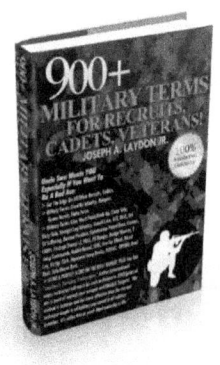

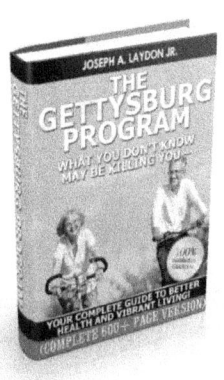

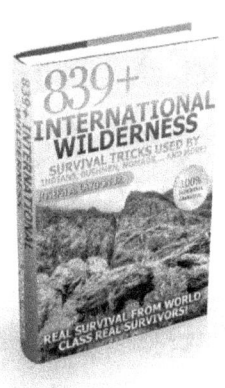

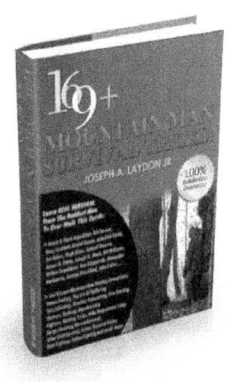

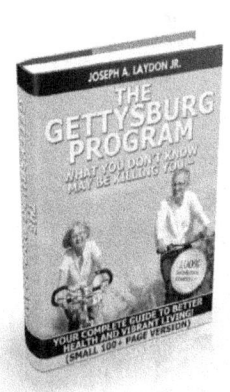

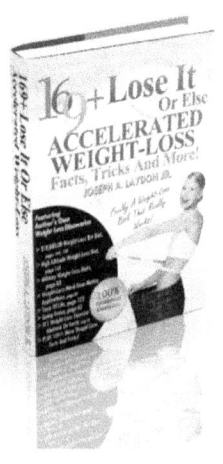

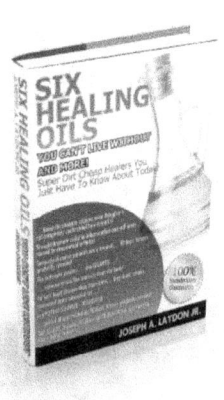

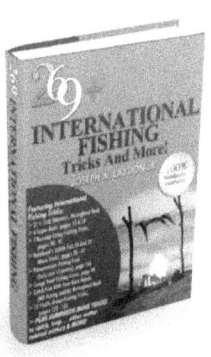

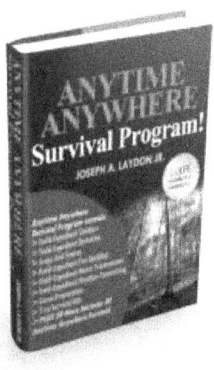

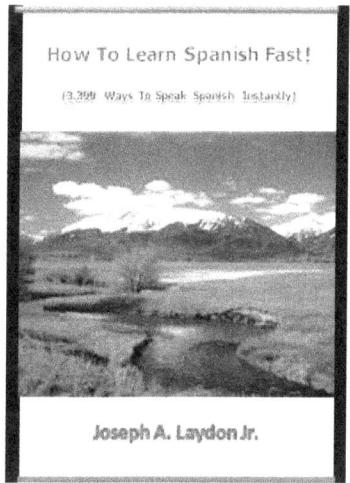

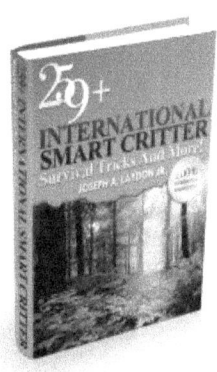

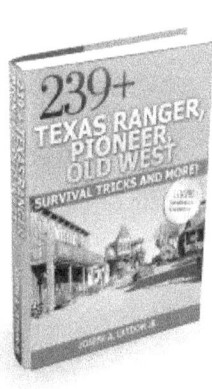

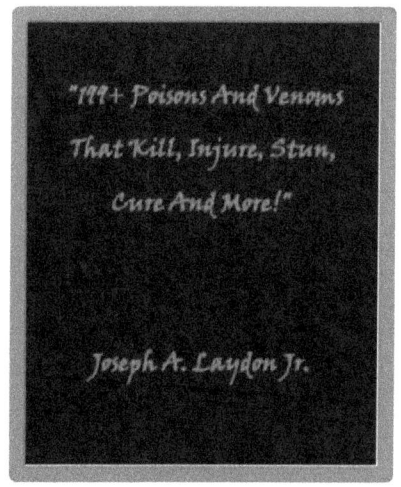

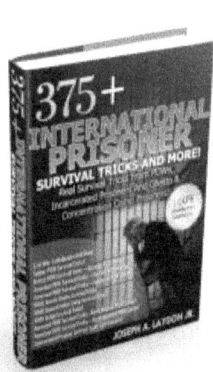

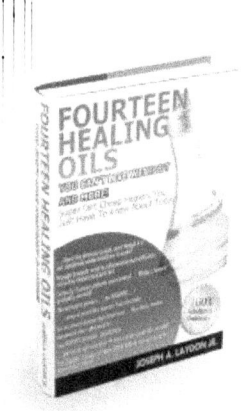

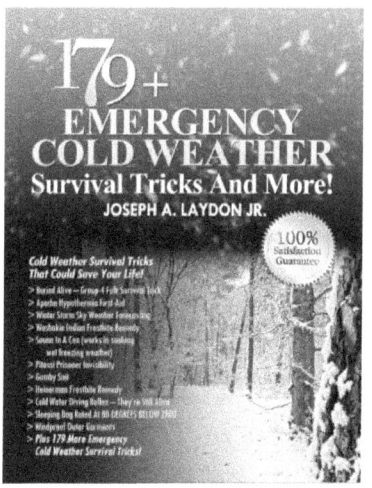

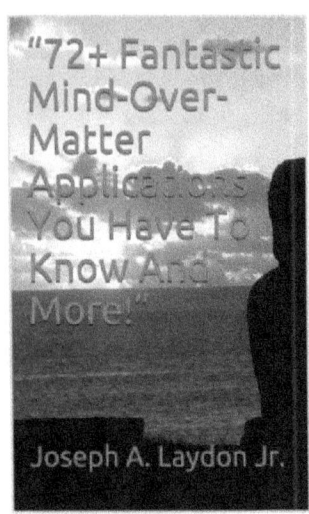

"72+ Fantastic Mind-Over-Matter Applications You Have To Know And More!"

Joseph A. Laydon Jr.

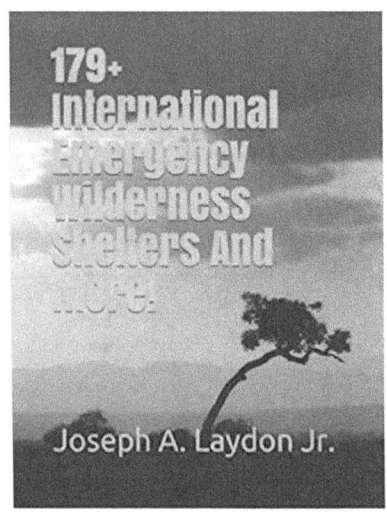

179+ International Emergency Wilderness Shelters And More!

Joseph A. Laydon Jr.

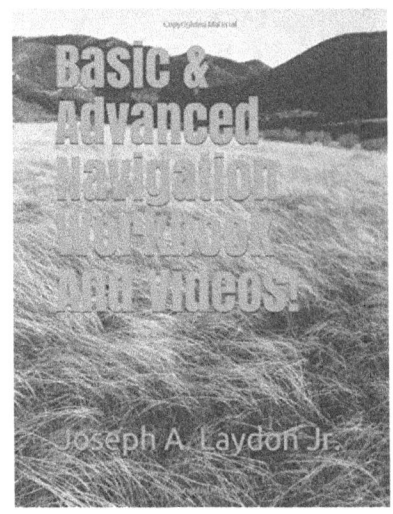

Basic & Advanced Navigation Methods And Videos!

Joseph A. Laydon Jr.

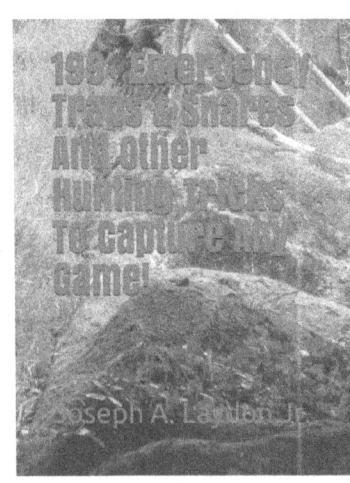

199+ Emergency Traps & Snares And Other Hunting Tactics To Capture Any Game!

Joseph A. Laydon Jr.

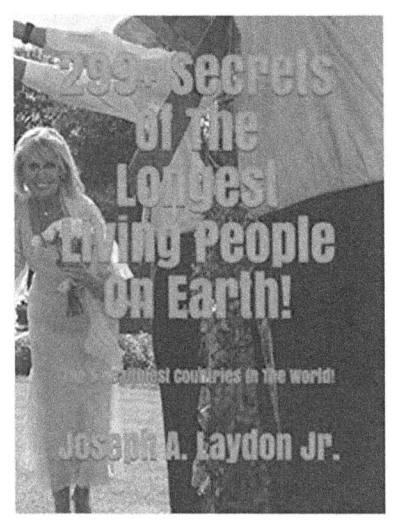

299+ Secrets Of The Longest Living People On Earth!

Joseph A. Laydon Jr.

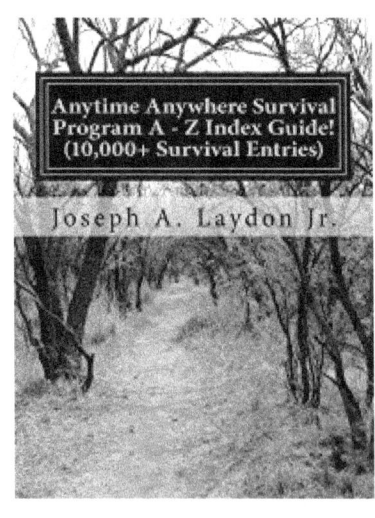

Anytime Anywhere Survival Program A - Z Index Guide! (10,000+ Survival Entries)

Joseph A. Laydon Jr.

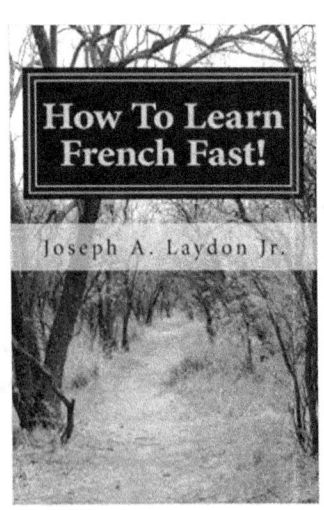

How To Learn French Fast!

Joseph A. Laydon Jr.

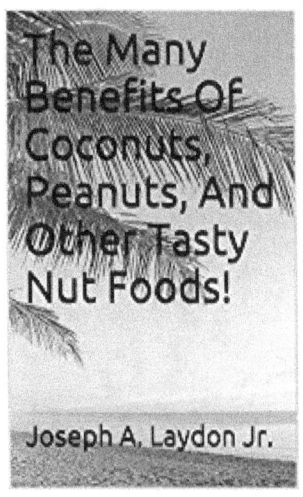

The Many Benefits Of Coconuts, Peanuts, And Other Tasty Nut Foods!

Joseph A. Laydon Jr.

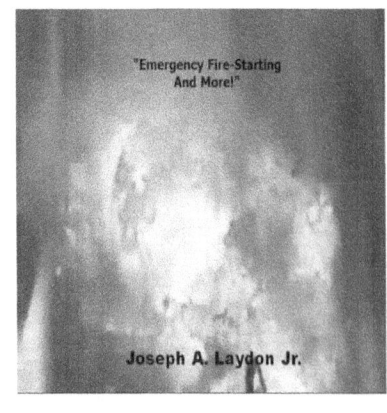

"Emergency Fire-Starting And More!"

Joseph A. Laydon Jr.

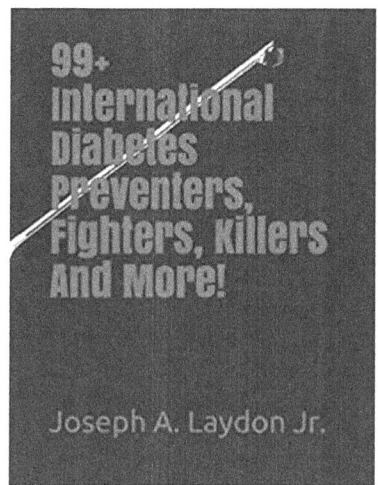
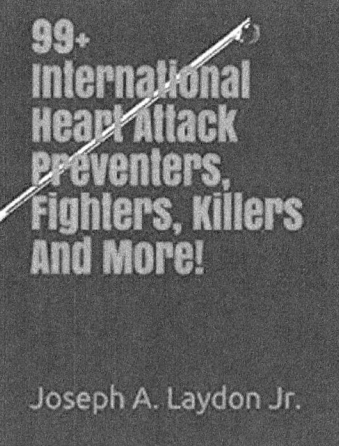
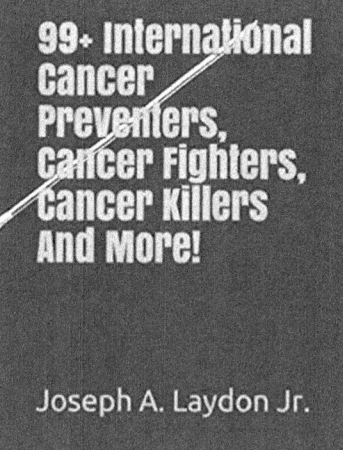

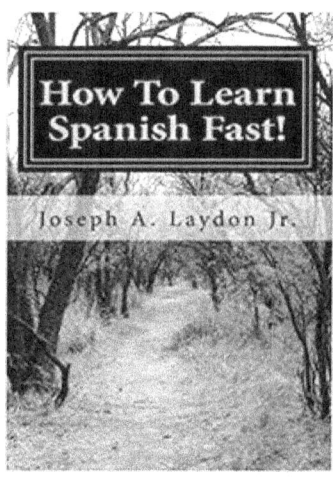
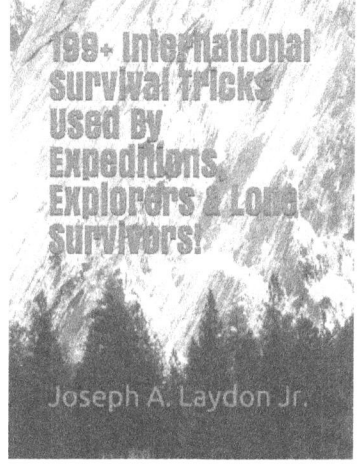
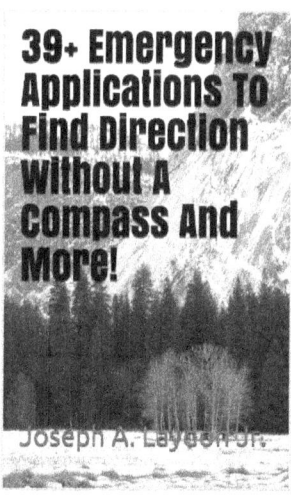

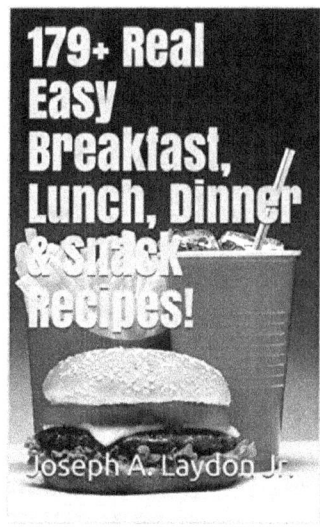
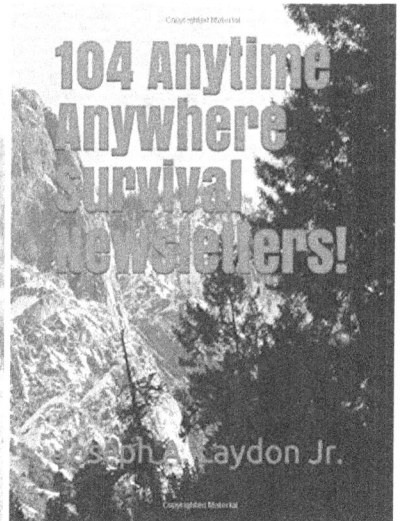

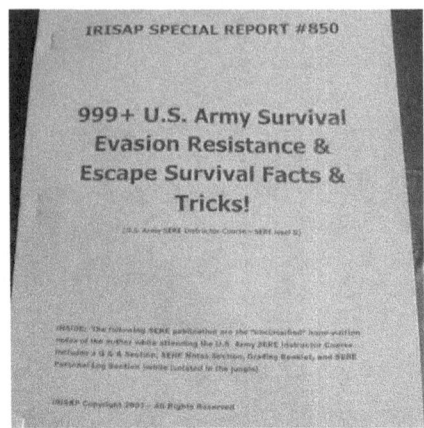

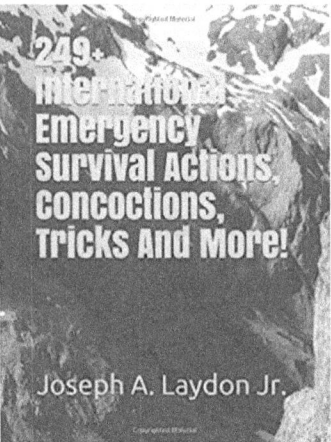

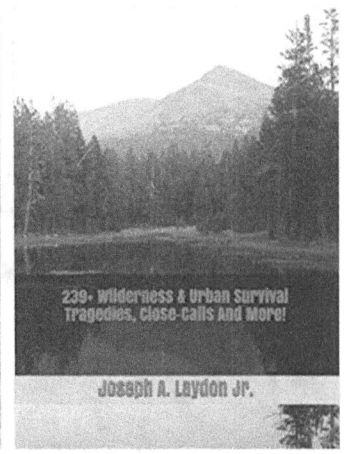

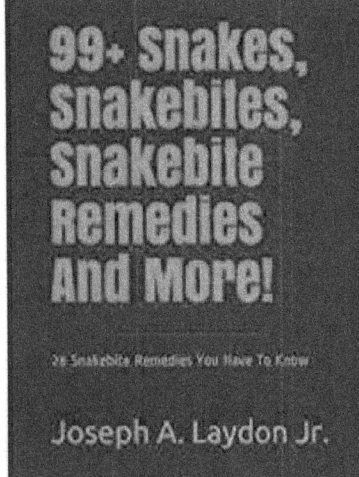

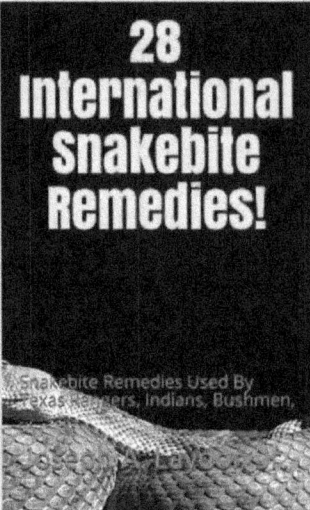

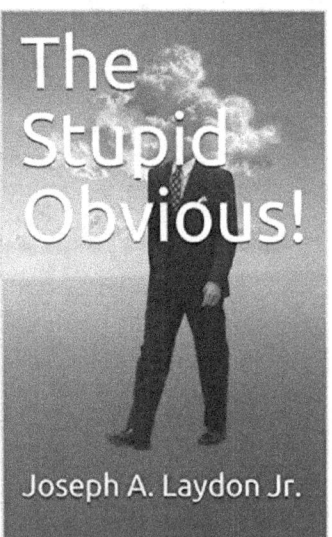

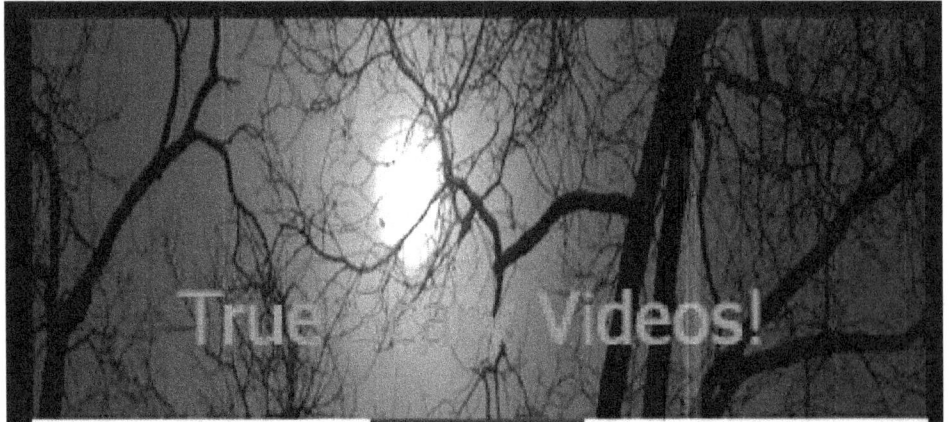

www.truescaryvideos.com

About The Author

Joseph A. Laydon Jr. (MSG (E-8) Retired United States Army - 18Z5V) is 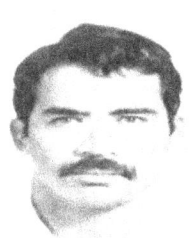 the author and owner of *Intensive Research Information Services And Products (IRISAP)*. Joseph is a well-qualified instructor in international wilderness survival and the other 03 Survivals he teaches (Health Survival, Crime Survival and Money Survival). He is a 20-year US Army veteran (Master Sergeant E-8 - 18Z5V) associated with all Special Operations units in the US military, as well as Special Ops units in the Mid-East and Central & South America.

He's a qualified SERE Instructor (Survival Evasion Resistance & Escape) and has **taught wilderness survival** at the college level for 03 years. He's a qualified instructor in basic & advanced pistol marksmanship, basic & advanced rifle marksmanship, CQB (Close Quarter Battle), basic & advanced cross-country navigation, basic mountaineering techniques, and self-defense. Since 1994, he's published many self-improvement Survival Programs, Survival Videos, SPECIAL Reports, Intelligence Reports, monthly Newsletters, **100+ Survival Books** (Kindle E-Books & Kindle Paperback Books) and more in the works.

He's an inventor, he *"sideways engineers"* new survival tricks that can SAVE YOUR LIFE! An example: On 17 August 2000 - 1417 hours, at Scott Lake, Scott AFB, IL, Joseph made international history! He is the 1st in the world to replicate the mysterious fires of Africa using a single drop of water! On 05 January 2001, he discovered how to start a life-saving fire in just 02-seconds using a beam of light from a flashlight in pitch black *"blind man"* darkness! On 06 April 2005 - 1810 hours, he invented delicious & tasty Solid Fuel Rolls and several Trail-Mix Cookies that are used as emergency foods and used as long-burning emergency fire-starting kindling.

And recently - **50+ MORE TOP SECRET INVENTIONS** of advanced & **ultra-advanced fire-starting** like starting EMERGENCY FIRE-STARTING using personal care products and first-aid products you already use like:

- Shampoo

- Toothpastes
- Mouthwashes
- Breath Drops & Breath Sprays
- Salves
- Ointments
- Over-The-Counter Medicines
- Drink Enhancement Products
- Other ingredients like your spit (saliva), your urination,...

See **www.survivalexpert.com/fire**

He also teaches Advanced Navigation (*Basic & Advanced Navigation Workbook And Videos* [includes Workbook, Videos, maps, protractors,…]) so you're ready Anytime Anywhere! Only from IRISAP and only for privileged IRISAP subscribers - YOU! See *Basic & Advanced Navigation Workbook And Videos* at **www.survivalexpertbooks.com/navigation**

Below is a sample of his military achievements & qualifications (**not in chronological order**) which reflect his unique & superior ability to teach basic, advanced & ultra-advanced survival applications, techniques and "tricks" that could help you AVOID serious killer survival threats as well as SAVE YOUR LIFE when you get in life or death situations. His trade secrets, Programs, and Videos are only offered to IRISAP subscribers-YOU!

- US Army Airborne School
- US Army Special Forces Qualification Course - SFQC (Green Beret)
- US Army Master Parachutist Wings
- Uruguayan Parachutist Wings
- British Parachutist Wings
- Kingdom of Jordan Parachutist Wings
- Expert Infantry Badge - EIB
- 82nd Airborne Division Recondo Course
- Adverse Weather Aerial Delivery System Tests - AWADS (01 of 386 volunteer paratroopers)
- US Army Special Forces Weapons Course (US & foreign pistols, submachineguns, assault rifles, rifles, machineguns, mortars, anti-tank weapons, anti-aircraft weapons,…)

- Weapons Armorer Course
- Indirect Fire Course (60mm, 81mm, & 4.2 inch *"four deuce"* mortars)
- Jumpmaster Course
- Basic French Language Course
- Combat Infantry Badge - CIB
- US Army Ranger Course
- Advanced Navigation Course
- Special Forces Sniper Course (02)
- Survival Evasion Resistance and Escape Instructor Course (SERE Level B)
- Wilderness Survival Instructor (College level - 03 years / 1991 - 1994)
- Rappell Master
- Fast Rope Master
- International Sniper Instructor
- International Close Quarter Battle (CQB) Instructor
- Participated In Multiple Combat Actions
- Special Forces Operations And Intelligence Course (O&I)
- Good Conduct Medal (06)
- Army Commendation Medal
- Army Achievement Medal (02)
- Meritorious Service Medal (02)
- Armed Forces Expeditionary Medal
- Letters Of Commendation (13)
- Letters Of Appreciation (08)
- Infantry Advanced NCO Course (11B)**
- Infantry Officer Basic Course **
- Military Intelligence Officer Basic Course **
- Held **SECRET** and **TOP SECRET Clearances** for 20+ years

** = These are military home study correspondence courses which took years to complete. This demonstrates Mr. Laydon's dedication to duty and desire to go beyond the training standards set by the US Army Special Forces. You won't find too many soldiers completing years of military home study courses on their own time off. This reflects the author's many superior Survival Products like this Survival Product.

Featured on FOX-2 (24 August 2000). Joseph now resides in Illinois. He offers products concerning Wilderness Survival, Health Survival, Crime Survival and Money Survival so to greatly enhance the lives of all IRISAP subscribers - YOU! Any questions, write to Joseph today.

Sincerely,
Joseph A. Laydon Jr. (IRISAP)
P.O. Box 48
Cutler, IL 62238-0048

You And Yours Have A Safe One
Anytime Anywhere,

Joseph A. Laydon Jr.

E-Mail: wwwsurvivalexpert@yahoo.com

E-Mail: josephlaydonjr@gmail.com

WEBSITES

- Main Website--------------------www.survivalexpertblog.com
- 50+ Survival Paperback Books-----www.survivalexpertblog.com/52-survival-books/
- 50+ Survival Kindle E-Books------www.survivalexpertblog.com/52-survival-books/
- Anytime Anywhere Survival--------www.anytimeanywheresurvival.com
- Weight-Loss---------------------www.loseitorelseweightloss.com
- True Scary Videos---------------www.truescaryvideos.com
- Exodus To Genesis (Fiction Book)-www.exodustogenesis.com
- **NEW** – 'Survival Expert Blog'--https://www.survivalexpertblog.com
- **NEW & IMPROVED** – *'Save My Life - Basic, Advanced And Ultra-Advanced Emergency Fire-Starting TOTAL Package'*
  https://www.survivalexpertblog.com/save-my-life-survival-program

IRISAP Copyright 2017 – All Rights Reserved

Take Notes

Take Notes

Take Notes

Take Notes

Take Notes

Take Notes

Take Notes

Take Notes

"More Heathy Books Worthy Of Your Attention!"

<u>THANK YOU, THANK YOU, THANK YOU for getting this Health Survival Book</u>. I want to let you know there are other Healthy Books that are worthy of your attention. I want to tell you, I am not a doctor nor am I qualified in any health profession. My job is I do research – *"Intensive Research."*. Here are some of my other 'health related' books that are worthy of your attention.

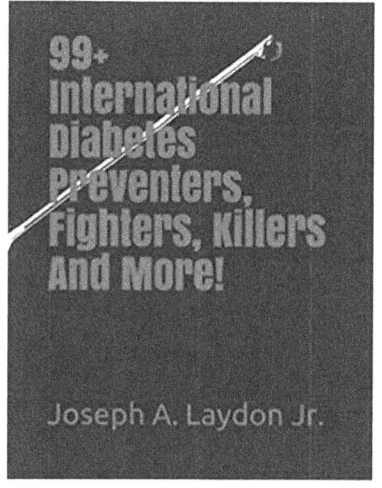 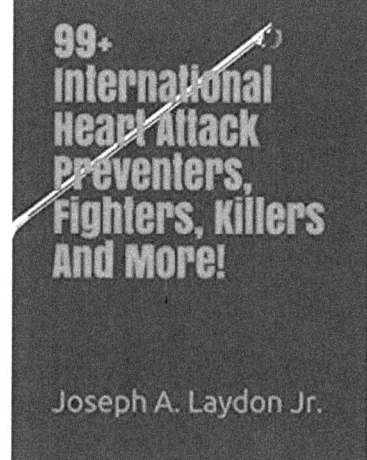 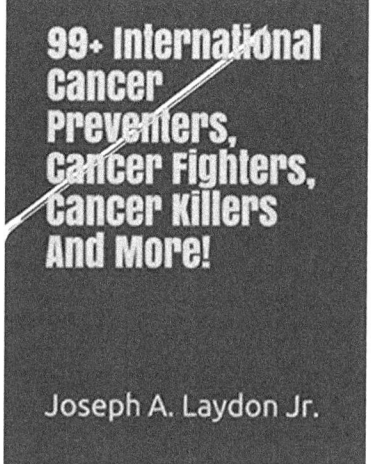

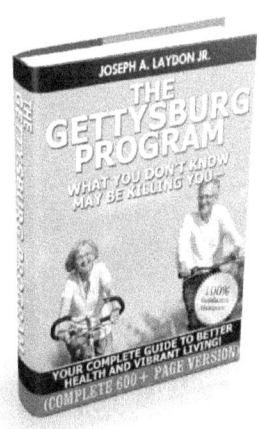 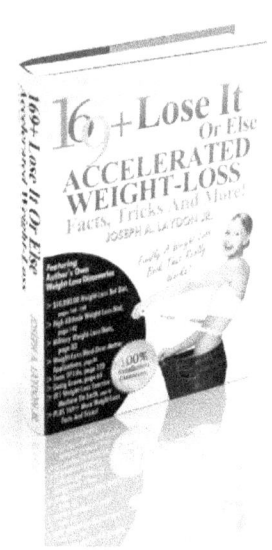 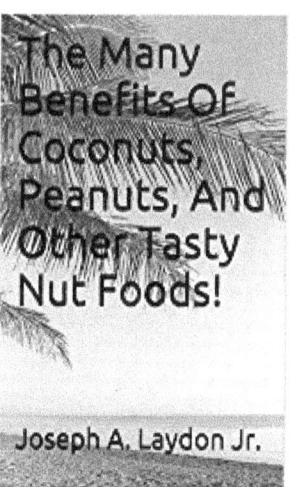

https://survivalexpertblog.com/52-survival-books/
(Paperback Books)

https://survivalexpertblog.com/52-survival-books/
(Kindle E-Books)